THE PSYCHOBIOLOGY OF CANCER

THE PSYCHOBIOLOGY OF CANCER

Automatization and Boredom in Health and Disease

Augustin M. de la Peña

Chief, Clinical Psychophysiology Laboratory
Audie L. Murphy Memorial Veterans Administration Hospital
and
University of Texas Medical School
Psychology Division, Department of Psychiatry

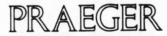

PRAEGER SPECIAL STUDIES • PRAEGER SCIENTIFIC
F. BERGIN PUBLISHERS

Library of Congress Cataloging in Publication Data

De la Peña, Augustin.
  The psychobiology of cancer.

  Bibliography: p. 175.
  Includes index.
  1. Carcinogenesis—Philosophy. 2. Cancer—Psychosomatic aspects. 3. Mind and body.
4. Diseases—Causes and theories of causation. 5. Boredom. I. Title. [DNLM: 1. Neo-
plasms—Etiology. 2. Psychophysiologic disorders. 3. Neoplasms—Psychology. QZ 202.
D338p]
  RC268.5.D44   616.99′4071   81-10110
  ISBN 0-03-062872-5
                                                              AACR2

All rights reserved
J.F. Bergin Publishers, Inc.
670 Amherst Road
South Hadley, Mass. 01075

Published in 1983 by Praeger Publishers
CBS Educational and Professional Publishing
A Division of CBS, Inc.
521 Fifth Avenue, New York, New York 10175 U.S.A.

0123456789   056   987654321

Printed in the United States of America

To
Colin Wilson, Charles Furst, and Jean Hamilton, contemporary
pioneers in the psychobiology of interest-boredom

Contents

Foreword

A large body of research in the combined fields of psychology, medicine, and the basic sciences lends support to the notion that cancer exists not as a cellular entity, but rather as a function of the total behavioral history of the organism. The breadth and comprehensiveness of this research is remarkably obscure, however, possibly because it emanates from scientists from numerous disciplines who do not, as a matter of course, communicate with one another professionally. The literature itself has been reviewed by several writers in some detail, with the usual intent to either provide support for or against the thesis that psychological factors are related to neoplastic development. The usual conclusion is that a relationship exists, but that the nature of the relationship is unclear.

De la Peña's treatise embarks on a most timely and necessary next phase in this research, i.e., theory building to provide a framework both for understanding previous findings and for guiding subsequent research. Without such a theoretical foundation many of the earlier studies are not only paradoxical, but so confusing that an uncomfortable aura of randomness exists when they are considered *in toto*. The notion of information underload/overload as presented in this book grants an order to the data which it has desperately lacked up to now.

Essentially, the author suggests that carcinogenesis can occur as a result not only of information overload but of information underload. He marshals the evidence for this position from a wide variety of resources, including biology, genetics, and physiology, as well as from multiple areas within psychology. De la Peña handles the multidisciplinary language beautifully, displaying the vast amount of information necessitated by a more holistic approach to the subject matter. Further, he proposes that subsequent research be less molecular, with an eye toward the identification of curvilinear relationships among etiological variables and the occurrence of carcinoma. That suggests a very different paradigm for treatment and research than now exists under the auspices of our current "war on cancer." Whether one chooses to agree with de la Peña's orientation will be, of course, a personal decision based on professional background and identification. What *is* certain is that the scholarly presentation will be sufficiently provocative to encourage new vistas.

Jeanne Achterberg
The University of Texas
Health Science Center at Dallas

Introduction

It is the business of the future to be dangerous.

The major advances in civilization are processes
that all but wreck the societies in which they occur.

A. N. Whitehead
Adventures in Ideas

Everyday experience and a little bit of introspection point out a paradox of contemporary western life. Technological developments in the physical sciences have released human beings from tedious, mind-numbing tasks, given them increasing control over the vicissitudes of nature, helped to eradicate certain kinds of illness and disease, and provided an unprecedented amount of freedom and leisure time. However, instead of monolithic progress toward a state of individual well-being, health, and realization of potential, as well as the continued discovery of marvels in technology, medicine, and society, we observe contradictory developments: the possibility of nuclear annihilation; accelerated war and violence, distrust, and paranoia toward self and society; an increasingly exploited, polluted, and overpopulated planet; a leisure society frantically involved in staying busy, struggling to stay awake or fall asleep, fighting feelings of boredom, depression, alienation, and spiritual dyspepsia; increasing rates of homicide, suicide, schizophrenia, neurosis, obesity, alcoholism, cardiovascular disease, and cancer.

Experience also acquaints us with the inadequacies of contemporary medicine and psychology in improving the human condition. At a time when advances in the physical sciences have given humankind mastery over many aspects of the environment, medicine and psychology continue to disappoint. The inadequacies of current health care practice are obvious: while there is no doubt that psychiatry is progressing as a discipline and a science, psychiatric patients continue to fill a major proportion of hospital beds; the long-term efficacy of psychotherapy and psychopharmacological treatments has yet to be demonstrated. Similarly, while medicine is spectacularly effective in the treatment of traumatic structural damage and infectious disease, it is marginally, if at all, effective in treating chronic degenerative diseases and life style problems such as drug addiction, obesity, alcoholism, and stress management. The predominant physical diseases of contemporary man such as cancer, cardiovascular disease, and pain syndromes remain stubbornly resistant to traditional medical intervention.

As a health science professional who has worked in medical schools and hospitals for a decade, I have had personal contact with the limitations and inadequacies of the current paradigm in the diagnosis and treatment of mental and physical disorders. From the problems and frustrations I experience in my own clinical (psychophysiological) work with sleep and stress disordered patients, from discussions with physicians who have intimate involvement and responsibility in our country's leading medical establishments, from recent reviews of national health care statistics suggesting the questionable contribution of medical advances and interventions to the decline of mortality in the United States (McKinlay and McKinlay, 1980), from thoughtful articles describing the progressive disillusionment with present day curative medicine (Saward and Sorenson, 1980)—from all of these sources, the message is clear: the current medical (mechanistic) approach to the management of health and disease, as practiced privately and in our most prestigious medical institutions, is inefficient and becoming increasingly discouraging for both patient and physician.

Recognizing the limitations of the current mechanistic-reductionistic approach to medicine, a growing number of individuals in health care delivery systems are endorsing a more holistic view of health and disease. However, the current holistic approach currently is without a guiding scientific framework for investigating the problem of mind (consciousness)—behavior (including health behavior) interrelations. Rather, current holistic approaches in most instances have adopted a mindless, nomethetic, cafeteria-style, behavioral approach to preventive medicine which is given to passing fads and general quackery. It is mindless in the sense that the behavioristic approach, based on learning theory and its principles, generally ignores mediating, biological (genetic), and cognitive variables. It is nomethetic because individual differences are largely ignored; it employs a cafeteria- style approach in that physicians and other health science practitioners generally prescribe changes in various aspects of behavior (diet, self-talk, relaxation exercises, physical exercise) depending mainly upon the availability of these resources in their armamentarium of expertise and facilities.

A similar dilemma characterizes the contemporary research enterprise in medicine, particularly in the cancer field. Since the discovery in the 1950s of the genetic importance of the nucleic acids, the largest share of the investment in cancer research has been in molecular approaches. However, while there have been striking advances in molecular biology and virology, including the isolation from human tumors of two specific tumor-associated viruses, there has been relatively little progress in understanding the nature of carcinogenesis. I suggest here that attempting to understand cancer exclusively from a molecular viewpoint fails to provide an adequate overview for guiding experimental work, i.e., principles derived from molecular studies lack sufficient scope to embrace the essential features of neoplasia. The paucity of general discussions of cancer in the literature during the past two decades is a testimony to this deficiency (Smith and Kenyon, 1973). What is advocated here is not so much a de-emphasis of molecular investigations of carcinogenesis, but rather an equal emphasis on a molar-synthetic approach to cancer. The living organism is a hierarchy of processes. Since the level of the genome is only one part of the hierarchical system, and no particular level is considered primary, other parts of the system are equally worthy of research investment and study.

My aim in writing this book is to offer a potentially more valid conceptual approach to the nature and etiology of health and disease, with a particular focus on cancer, based on a novel synthesis of knowledge emerging from the study of control systems (cybernetics) and information theory, and recent advances in neuropsychology, cognitive-developmental psychophysiology, and physics. My approach suggests that contemporary models of the psychobiology of cancer, indeed of health-disease broadly considered, are of limited utility because they employ an obsolete paradigm to aid in theory construction and data gathering. The current dominant biomedical paradigm is based on a mechanistic, reductionistic, Newtonian world-view which is inconsistent with developments in contemporary physics, information science, and cognitive psychology. This is not a new idea. It has been articulated by increasing numbers of scientists, health care professionals and health care critics (Bateson, 1979; Battista, 1977; Capra, 1977; Engel, 1977; Illich, 1976; Moser, 1977; Pelletier, 1978, 1979; Toffler, 1980).

The novelty of the book is the construction of a theoretical framework which is built upon premises consistent with twentieth century psychology, physics, and information science; the approach offers a new way of thinking about the etiology and nature of cancer, as well as health and disease broadly considered.

The principal arguments are as follows:

1. Increments in experience, including phylogenetic "experience," are associated with increments in automatization of information processing. Automatization refers to an efficient decrease in the amount of sensory information necessary to construct a repeated perceptual event. Phenomenologically, the term implies a reduction of consciousness or awareness of stimulus configurations and contingencies one acquires as a result of past experience with stimuli; this relative lack of awareness is associated with the experience of boredom.

2. Automatization of information processing makes possible the development of an impressive repertoire of perceptual, cognitive, and motor skills which lie at the core of what we call intelligence; that is, once an activity or stimulus is repeatedly experienced and becomes

automatized, it can be performed by some lower-order, less flexible cognitive subprogram. This leaves room in the central processor of the brain to acquire *new* information and skills; with practice, the new skills become automatized allowing new learning to take place, and so on.

3.   Increases in automatization are associated with the experience of boredom and/or ennui. This is because the more experienced the structure, the greater its ability to predict environmental stimulus configurations and contingencies, since a relatively large amount of the information is already encoded in structural and memorial processes. The consequence is a relatively low intensity of consciousness and/or relatively low information flow upon exposure to ordinary sensory environments. The experience of boredom is the phenomenological correlate of this low-intensity state.

4.   Structures have optimal ranges/rates of information flow. Information flow above or below this range is associated with the experience of "stress" or "anxiety." The more experienced the structure, the greater the need for information-flow-enhancing activity for organized function (behavioral, perceptual, etc.) of the structure, and the greater the probability of information underload (boredom) stress. This is because for experienced structures most of the information in ordinary environments is already encoded in memory and hence effects a relatively low rate of information flow relative to that obtaining for less experienced structures. The relatively low information-flow rate is rectified by information-augmenting perceptual, behavioral, and somatic activity.

5.   Excessive automatization generally obtains when highly experienced cognitive structures interact with environments which are relatively poor in terms of sensory and/or ideational information. Excessive automatization effects a decrease in the amount of information flow for the cortex to *sub-optimal* levels for organized cortical function.

6.   The excessively automatized (bored) brain has a variety of mechanisms for rectifying sub-optimal information flow levels to higher, optimal levels. Some of these mechanisms are expressed as behavioral, perceptual or cognitive "creativity," as in the production of original works in art and science. Other mechanisms seem to be expressed as perceptual, behavioral and/or somatic processes which are labeled as disease, illness, or disorder by the medical establishment. In general, then, the excessively automatized (bored) brain modulates information flow to higher, more optimal levels by promoting perceptions and behaviors, including illness behaviors, which serve a de-automatizing role.

7.   I suggest that many (but not all) of the major psychological, behavioral and somatic disorders which afflict contemporary adulthood humans, represent the manifestation of covert compensatory, homeostatic attempts by the excessively automatized (bored) brain to rectify its own sub-optimal rate of information processing. These attempts at optimal cortical information flow, while often adaptive for the

individual brain over the short-term, are often deleterious over the long term to the integrity of supra- (the individual, family, society) or sub-(organs, cells) structures in the hierarchy of structures in nature.

8.   A minority of the illnesses and disorders which afflict contemporary Western adulthood man are associated with excessive *de*-automatization of information processing for the brain. Excessive de-automatization obtains when there is a mismatch between the optimal information load of minimally experienced structures (low) and the amount of information in the environment (high); it occurs predominantly in the early childhood state, in various forms of mental retardation, and in certain adults who in an attempt to de-automatize, bite off more uncertainty than they can handle with existing cognitive structures.   In these cases, the illness and disorder represent a heterostatic de-automatizing process which is out of control and which hastens demise of the organism.

9.   Finally, it is suggested that a process similar to, if not identical with, optimal information load mismatch is experienced by sub- and supra-cortical structures in the hierarchy of structures in nature.   Sub-CNS mismatch considerations play a major role in determining the site of somatic disorder.   Supra-CNS mismatch is posited to guide evolution towards the development of mechanisms (sex, death, imagination, etc.) which increase the variety, and thus the information in nature, as nature gains increments in experience and becomes increasingly automatized.

Evidence is presented to support the view that contemporary society's health problems are created by the same process that is responsible for society's greatest achievements. Automatization of attention is the process which is central in the genesis of man's greatest artistic, scientific and behavioral achievements, and his most serious, life-threatening problems. A review of the literature suggests that excessive automatization of attention and its phenomenological sequela of boredom is a primary etiological element in a broad range of so-called mental, behavioral, and physical diseases, including some forms of cancer, some varieties of cardiovascular disease, some varieties of alcoholism, schizophrenia, suicide, acts of impulsive violence, gambling and other risk-taking behaviors, various sleep disorders, and a broad spectrum of miscellaneous "minor" physical disorders, such as some types of hypoglycemia, arthritis, allergy, and pain syndromes.

In addition, evidence is presented which suggests the possibility that automatization of information processing occurs not only for the brain, but at other levels within the hierarchy of structures in nature, i.e. in cells, organs.   Thus, I have suggested the interrelatedness of many processes in nature which are considered as separate and distinct by present day approaches.

The book is organized into ten chapters.   Chapter I gives an overview of current theory and research on cancer, emphasizing the breadth of environmental and biological-structural variables known to be associated with cancer. Chapter 2 describes some of the underlying premises of my developmental-structural approach which relate to concepts such as cognitive structure, information, and optimal information load. Other underlying premises related to the concepts of automatization, system, and emergence are treated in Chapter 3. Experimental support for the mismatch hypothesis of carcinogenesis is provided in Chapter 4. Chapter 5 continues the exposition of support for the hypothesis, highlighting correlational, non-experimental literature.

Support for mismatch theory from studies of non-CNS phenomena is outlined in Chapter 6. The explanatory utility, predictions, and implications of the mismatch hypothesis are described in Chapter 7; particular emphasis is given to the implications for preventive treatment aspects. Chapter 8 points out the extension of mismatch theory to a broad range of health phenomena, suggesting that the etiology of many somatic, behavioral, and mental disorders may be conceptualized from the same vantage point. In Chapter 9 mismatch theory is applied to a broad range of sleep disorders. Chapter 10 describes the current ascendance of the systems approach in scientific research, the ascendance of consciousness as the central problem in physical and psychological science, and the critical need for a valid metaphysics and epistemology of nature, if nature is to continue to evolve.

The book is ultimately a synthesis of the thought and work of many individuals. The greatest intellectual debt is owed Jean Piaget, Colin Wilson, Charles Furst, John Battista, and the late Ludwig von Bertalanffy. There are many other theorists and workers from whom ideas and attitudes were collated, and acknowledgment must of necessity take the form of references in the text.

The first draft of the present book was completed in 1974, during my first year at the University of Texas Health Science Center and the Audie Murphy Memorial Veterans Hospital in San Antonio. Alvin Burstein and Kenneth Gaarder were helpful, at that stage, in pointing out sections in need of clarification. A second draft received encouraging comments from Robert Ornstein, Sara Hoeback, Herbert Weiner, Jean Hamilton, Larry Gaupp, Colin Wilson, Charles Furst and William Estes. In 1978-79, Arthur Koestler, Jackie Lanum and Hans Selye read the draft and contributed favorable comments and encouragement. In 1980, John Battista provided positive feedback.

This book has been helped along the way by many other individuals. Fleming Henry James and Charles Chaplin assembled most of the bibliography and did much of the library work. Patricia Riley and Ellen Hanks of the medical school library staff coordinated the task of reference verification. Ed Kollar, Alvin Burstein and Robert Leon provided encouragement and support. Catherine Gary, Sara Hoeback and Annette Richardson provided invaluable editorial assistance. Sharon Tumlinson typed the first draft, and Carl Erickson typed the final draft. I am indebted to clinical research associates Doug McDaniel, Donald Mayfield, Richard Flickinger, George Garza, and Joe De Cesare, whose talents and competence in various aspects of clinical psychophysiology allowed me time to complete this book. However, the actual writing and typing of the manuscript has not been done at any government expense.   Finally, special thanks to Peggy Seeger and Jenna Schulman for editorial refinements.

Chapter 1 Toward a Holistic Approach to Carcinogenesis

Whole sight; or all the rest is desolation.

John Fowles
Daniel Martin

INTRODUCTION

The Concept Of Paradigm

The term paradigm refers to a set of basic assumptions or premises that underlie a theory. Frequently, these assumptions are not recognized or made explicit. Since assumptions both define and limit a theory's scope, it is important to recognize these basic premises in theory construction. For example, given the assumptions of the mechanistic paradigm, psychic phenomena are generally dismissed as mental aberrations because such phenomena cannot be handled within a mechanistic conceptual framework (Battista, 1977).

A number of authors (Harman, 1974; Laszlo, 1972; Lifton, 1975; Sutherland, 1973) have implied that a new paradigm shift is occurring in most fields of science. The newly emerging paradigm is called "holistic" and shows promise of supplanting the mechanistic paradigm which has dominated science until recently as the best foundation for a metatheory of the physical, biological, psychological and social sciences.

In order to define and delimit the holistic approach, it is first helpful to contrast its assumptions with those of the vitalistic and mechanistic approaches. Paradigms are defined by the way in which they answer the three fundamental questions of the philosophy of science (Battista, 1977). What is the nature of reality (metaphysics)? How do we acquire knowledge (epistemology)? What accounts for change and stability (dynamics or means of explanation)?

Vitalistic, Mechanistic and Holistic Paradigms

The vitalistic paradigm assumes that the universe is divided into a vital, living force and a mechanical physical world. The vital force is

1

directional and purposeful; it is nonlocalizable and forms the basis of all life. Dualism also characterizes the mechanistic paradigm, but it divides the world into matter-energy and space-time. The holistic paradigm views the universe monistically, as one interconnected system. Living and nonliving, matter and energy, space and time are all conceptualized as transformations within a hierarchically ordered unity (Battista, 1977).

In the vitalistic paradigm, knowledge is gained through experience. The validity of the vital force is self-evident because we can feel its pull. The mechanistic paradigm assumes that truth is objective, it resides in a world external to us, and can be analyzed and understood by empirical methodology which alters the world with mechanical forces and measures the results. One understands a phenomenon when it can be analyzed in terms of a mechanical law based on the fundamental concepts of mass, energy, space and time. Newtonian physics represents the culmination of this approach.

In the holistic paradigm, truth exists in interaction between an observer and an observed; it involves both inner experience and external verification. Verification obtains through modeling. A model of the phenomenon is created and one attempts to determine if the properties of the model match the properties of the phenomenon. Thus explanation occurs via isomorphic analogy at the same order of complexity as the phenomenon to be explained instead of making reference to some higher order (vitalistic) or lower order (mechanistic) force (Battista, 1977).

Vitalism assumes that a passive, inert, and unmoving universe is impelled to change only through the action of an inherently active and purposeful vital force. The mechanistic paradigms view matter as passively driven by a mechanical force in a totally determined manner. Thus both vitalistic and mechanistic paradigms use energy as an explanatory concept: in vitalism, the force is outside of space and operates in time; in mechanism, the force is temporal, linear and dimensional. In contrast, holism views stability as the maintenance of the form of a system. Form is maintained because it is the result of the abiding structure or transformation matrix of the system, not because the energy-matter components of the system remain the same. That is, the human body maintains its form despite energy transformation within it. Change is viewed as a transformation of the system as the result of information processing; change refers to the reorganization of a set of mutually dependent, probabilistic variables which have "emergent" properties (Battista, 1977).

Emergence of the Holistic Paradigm in Medicine

In *The Structure of Scientific Revolutions,* Kuhn (1962) points out that every dominant paradigm eventually moves to the limits of its methodologies and ceases to be creative. As these limits are approached, there is an increasing body of information that it cannot incorporate and alternative paradigms come to the fore. Among the scientific revolutions described are the study of astronomy after Copernicus and the study of mechanics after Newton's *Principia* (Pelletier, 1979).

Medicine, based on Newtonian physics, has adhered for some time now to a mode of scientific inquiry with inherent assets and often unacknowledged limitations. Its central assumption has been that the whole can be understood through a fine analysis of its parts and ultimately the whole can be synthesized from knowledge of the parts. Such an approach focuses increasingly on minute parts of biological processes and generally has systematically excluded psychological and psychosocial variables. This relatively molecular approach has led to considerable progress and is consistent with seventeenth through nineteenth century science and philosophy. However, it is becoming increasingly evident that to limit all research and clinical applications to such a paradigm is no longer tenable. In fact, it is anachronistic to twentieth-century science and philosophy (Pelletier, 1979).

An orientation has emerged in health care which has been labeled "holistic medicine"—holistic derives from the Greek *holos* meaning whole. At the core of holistic medicine is the recognition that each state of health and disease requires a consideration of all contributing factors, physical-biological, psychological, environmental, etc. The holistic approach is inimical. to the prevailing reductionist model which seeks linear cause-and-effect relationships, whether based upon unconscious conflicts (as in psychoanalysis) or in aberrant molecular structures (as in molecular biology).

As pathology is examined with ever-increasing specialization, the major crises in contemporary medicine are for the most part overlooked. There is little need to search obscure journals or to depend on the most vocal spokesmen of the holistic approach for a constructive critique of the current malaise in medicine. In point of fact, some of the most articulate spokesmen on the limits of modern medicine are within the system itself. A recent article by F. J. Ingelfinger (1977), former editor of the *New England Journal of Medicine,* points out these limits.

> Let us assume that 80 percent of patients have either self-limited disorders or conditions not improvable, even by modern medicine. The physicians' actions, unless harmful, will therefore not affect the basic course of such conditions. In slightly over 10 percent of cases, however, medical intervention is dramatically successful, whether the surgeon repairs bones or removes stones, the internist uses antibiotics or palliative measures (e.g., insulin, Vitamin B_{12}) appropriately, or the pediatrician eliminates a food that an enzyme deficient infant cannot absorb or metabolize. But, alas, in the final 9 percent, give or take a point or two, the doctor may diagnose or treat inadequately, or he may just have

bad luck. Whatever the reason, the patient winds up with iatrogenic problems. So the balance of accounts ends up marginally on the positive side of zero.

Critics of the holistic approach are quick to impugn its scientific underpinnings or to point out that there is inadequate research evidence to document its effectiveness. Holists answer that the concept "scientific" should be revised to encompass non-linear notions of causality as described by general systems theory. They also point out that, although supporting research is inherently limited at this point primarily because it was started only a few years ago, there are nevertheless substantial clinical research trials where a holistic approach to preventive medicine has been evaluated and found to be demonstrably effective in reducing incidences of disease through preventive education (Harrington et al, 1977; Farquhar et al, 1977).

Moreover, the underlying epistemology of holistic medicine is consistent with *twentieth* century science and philosophy. Emerging from quantum physics and its philosophical implications is a new point of view wherein "the universe is no longer seen as a machine made up of a multitude of objects, but rather as a harmonious 'organic' whole whose parts are only defined through their interrelations" (Capra, 1977).

The physics of subatomic particles has thrust upon science the necessity of revising and extending previous concepts of reality. Quantum physics suggests two major revisions of significance for the development of a holistic approach to medicine. One is that subatomic particles do not exist as objects fixed in a specific space and time; rather objects exhibit "tendencies to exist" (Heisenberg, 1958), or as Stapp (1971) has amplified, this tendency or probability to exist does not refer to things, but rather to interconnections. An object "observed" at the quantum level is not an identifiable object, but rather an intermediate system dependent upon the preparation of the experiment and the subsequent means of measurement. Pelletier (1979: 26) describes the dilemma confronting contemporary medicine succinctly:

> Interactions of a quantum nature are of subtle energies that do not conform to Newtonian physics. Just as the physicist approaches the limits of New-tonian physics when dealing with subtle energy systems, biomedical researchers confront these same limits and need to revise their long standing neglect of psychological and psychosocial energies. Just as properties of quantum objects cannot be defined independently of preparation and measurement, people cannot be separated from their context and interaction with others.

A second revision is that the quantum perspective implies fundamentally different concepts of etiology relative to the Newtonian model. In the latter, disease taxonomy moves in a sequence of distinct stages: symptoms, groups of symptoms, syndromes, and finally an identifiable disease with a specific pathogenesis and a specific, rational treatment to follow (Fabrega, 1972, 1975). While such an approach has merit, it often may not hold up in actual practice. Moreover, as Engel (1977) has noted, it has a major defect in its logic. Ultimately, the approach is based upon the identification of the smallest isolable causative component, e.g., a specific bacteria or virus. As Pelletier notes (1979: 27) it is not at all clear that such an initial causative agent is applicable in any of the noninfectious afflictions of contemporary man. Engel (1977: 130) remarked:

> Thus the presence of the biochemical defect of diabetes or schizophrenia at best defines a necessary but not a sufficient condition for the occurrence for the human experience of the human disease, the illness. More accurately, the biochemical defect constitutes but one factor among many, the complex interaction of which ultimately may culminate in active disease or manifest illness.

In the current medical model, the presence of an abnormality vis-à-vis an objective diagnostic test is regarded as a specific criterion for a disorder. However, a laboratory test may be positive and yet the disorder not be evident (Engel, 1969). For example, diabetes is a disorder with clear diagnostic indications, but the extent to which an individual manifests physical or psychological impairment due to a deficiency of insulin depends upon numerous psychosocial influences.

The holistic approach takes a phenomenological view of disease and sees it as a neutral occurrence in an individual's lifetime. Ultimately, whether the disease is manifested or not, or whether its course is positive or negative, depends in part on the patient's cognitive interpretation of his illness, i.e., how the patient integrates the problem within the framework of his or her own structure of beliefs.

Optimum health is *not* mutually exclusive of periods of severe disease. A common observation is that individuals emerge from periods of profound psychological and physical pathology to function at higher levels of health than their previous norm (Perry, 1962). An extreme example occurs in the diagnosis of cancer (Pelletier, 1979). A critical period occurs between the first diagnosis and the time when the patient returns for further evaluation. Psychological reactions vary from deep depression to rampant anxiety to a determination to seize the opportunity and initiate positive life changes regardless of the final prognosis.[1]

Finally, not only is it possible for a causative agent to be present in the absence of disease, but it is also equally possible that a disorder be manifest without an attendant aberration at the biochemical level. White et al (1961), for example, studied the hospital admissions records of 1,000 adults per month over a four-year period in the United States and England; admissions varied with age, sex, and the seasons.   White concluded that entry into medical care systems apparently depends not only upon the "mechanisms" of disease," but also upon the "social, psychologic, cultural, economic, informational, administrative, and organizational factors that inhibit and facilitate access to and delivery of the best contemporary health care to individuals and communities" (1961: 890-891).

Numerous other concepts derived from relativity theory and quantum mechanics bear directly upon research concerning the role of "mind" in health and disease and the development of holistic medicine. These have been reviewed beautifully by Pelletier (1978) in *Toward a Science of Consciousness* and will be discussed in more detail in Chapter 10 of this book.   It will suffice to say here that intrapsychic and psychosocial factors influencing health and disease do not exist as identifiable "objects" in the obsolete (Newtonian) epistemology of medicine and hence have been relegated second class status in contemporary medicine's purely biomedical approach to health care.

In keeping with the holistic orientation and its underpinnings in twentieth century science and philosophy, this book seeks to develop a *principia* for the understanding of health and disease, with a focus on cancer.   The remainder of this chapter will present an overview of current theory and research on carcinogenesis.   The terms "cancer" and "carcinogenesis" are defined, and major characteristics of cancer cells are described.   The bulk of the chapter attempts to provide the reader with a bird's eye view of the broad range of biological, psychological, and environmental variables which are known to be associated with cancer.   The aim is not to be exhaustive, definitive and comprehensive, but to provide the reader a view of the forest (a description of the trees is deferred to later chapters).

CURRENT THEORY AND RESEARCH ON CANCER

The term cancer is defined, in this book, as a large variety of abnormal cellular growth and dispersion patterns, all characterized by cells growing when and where they should not, so that tissue (and subsequently, organismic) organization and homeostasis is threatened or weakened. The term carcinogenesis will refer to causative factors in cancer (tumor) induction and to their modes of action and thus comprises both the etiology and the pathogenesis of the disease.

Some Characteristics of Cancer Cells

Cancer cells are the progeny of normal cells.   Almost all types of differentiated cells—skin, kidney, nerve, etc.—can be transformed into cancer cells. Contiguous masses of cancer cells, called tumors, have great variation in rate of growth and extent of invasiveness. Malignant tumors grow rapidly and explosively, quickly spread through an organism, and invade a variety of normal tissues, leading inevitably to death. Benign tumors exhibit minimal growth rate, remain at the location where they arise, exist for years or even decades, and often are not harmful to the organism. Tumors also are classified along structural-morphological lines. Sarcomas are tumors of the connective or supporting tissues, bones, muscles, or nerves. Carcinomas are tumors of epithelial tissue, such as the breast, prostate, lung, and skin.

A cancer cell *cannot* be distinguished from a normal cell simply because it is constantly dividing (Watson, 1970). In mature animals, many normal cells are in constant growth and division to replace the large numbers that die each day (von Bertalanffy, 1960). Other normal cells, usually quiescent, suddenly begin to divide after the appearance of a specific hormone, and continue as long as the hormone is present. A cancer cell may not need the hormone stimulus, or it may require less hormone before commencing division. One useful distinction between normal and cancer cells is that the latter are less responsive to the normal control devices which cause cells not to divide (Watson, 1970). Normal cells are able to recognize one another when, in the formation of tissue, they come together, transmit information and cease to divide. One cell recognizes its neighbor's "personal space." The cancer cell, in contrast, is anarchistic. It divides regardless of neighboring cells and penetrates other tissue to establish colonies.

A crucial feature of a tumor is that it grows progressively in size (Berenblum, 1974). It never reaches growth equilibrium, the rate of cell division which is balanced by the rate of cell death. A disturbed growth equilibrium, and not simply rapid normal growth as in fetal development, is the characteristic of cancer. (An increase in mitotic rate, however, can exacerbate the effect by providing greater scope for the disequilibrium to express itself.)

Apart from differences that may exist between one tumor and another, there is also considerable variation among individual tumor cells. Even more striking is the erratic spatial relationship of the cells to one another (Berenblum, 1974). The more malignant a tumor, the greater the degree of tissue disorganization. In extreme forms of malignancy, the pattern may be entirely chaotic, and it is impossible to identify the cell type of origin. This condition, called anaplasia, is the morphological expression of the functional disturbances characteristic of malignancy which expresses itself in three ways (Berenblum, 1974): (1) a lower level of cell differentiation; (2) variation in size, shape and staining properties of the individual cells and their nuclei, as well as the presence of abnormal cell types; and (3) varying degrees of disorientation of the cells in relation to one another, expressive of diminished organization at the tissue level.

Some Characteristics of Carcinogenesis

Clinical knowledge of carcinogenesis covers almost two centuries of inquiry, with experimental research in animals beginning about sixty years ago.   Yet a satisfactory synthesis of the broad range of knowledge on the subject still has not been constructed.   The factors involved in the conversion from the normal to the cancerous state appear more complex than those found in other disease processes.   For example, in an inflammatory or degenerative disease, there are a rather limited number of etiological factors.   In cancer, by contrast, there are close to a thousand known chemical carcinogens, many physical carcinogens (e.g., X-rays, certain metals and plastic sheets), and certain viruses which may cause the disease, as well as modifying factors which may influence it.

In many forms of carcinogenesis, the beginning of the cancer process is apparently a change within the hereditary material (DNA) of the cell—a mutation.   However, not all mutations can be equated with cancer, necessarily lead to cancer, nor are inevitably irreversible (Richards, 1972).   There seem to be at least three steps in carcinogenesis (Richards, 1972).   Initially, the cancer may be dormant; the processes of cell growth and differentiation are only mildly at variance with their normal state.   But if the initiation process is followed by a process influenced by another agent, the neoplastic (cancer) cells grow from a dormant to a visible state. This second step is called promotion.   Finally, the process may continue and become irreversible.   But since the first step does not necessarily lead to cancer, if the second step fails to occur, the third and definitive step will not be attained.   In other words, the initial change in the hereditary structure may not be permanent or irreversible.   This concept of reversibility explains the well-established observation of regression in certain tumor growths.

One unusual feature of carcinogenesis is its biological expression of the process and the factors involved in it, which vary considerably with the tissue affected (Berenblum, 1974).   In mammary carcinogenesis the factors implicated are extremely varied, with viral, hormonal, and other components operating alone or interacting with specific carcinogenic factors.   But in other forms of cancer viral and hormonal involvement are less evident or even absent.

The usual explanation is that cancer is not a single entity, but represents a wide range of independent diseases comparable, say, to the many inflammatory diseases which are clinically distinct but pathologically related according to the micro-organism responsible. Nevertheless, it is generally assumed that there is also a basic unity for all forms of carcinogenesis despite the apparent diversity of mechanisms (Berenblum, 1974).

A new individual cell develops by a process of continuous cell division in which parts of a system having the same function and structure increase in size or number.   Since a size change usually precedes mitotic division, which in turn is necessary for the laying down of a discontinuity, growth is probably a more primary feature of development than is differentiation, in which some cells become blood, others liver, etc. (Thompson, 1968).   In the cancer cell, the procedure seems to reverse. As the tumor grows, the cells revert to an unspecialized, primitive, undifferentiated state in which growth rather than differentiation dominates (Baumler, 1968). Corroborating this notion, Wu (1973) concludes that the cancer cell reacquires the control mechanisms which prevailed early in the life of the organism; this reversion of some of the regulatory apparatus in the cancer cell to that in the prenatal stage of development is considered an essential mechanism in carcinogenesis.[2] Intercellular communication of information exists between adjacent normal epithelial cells via junctional complexes. Cancer cells are characterized by a lack of intercellular communication; they also lack junctional complexes (Dowben, 1971). This lack is probably associated with the cancer cell's inability to recognize its neighbor's "territory." The cell continues to grow and is deficient in "contact inhibition" (Watson, 1970).

Variables Influencing Carcinogenesis

A brief survey of the variables should aid in understanding current hypotheses of carcinogenesis and in recognizing their limitations.

Environmental Variables

Environment variables shown to be associated with carcinogenesis include specific properties of certain chemicals, physical agents, and the modulating influence of psychological, physical and psychophysiological stress.

CHEMICALS. Atmospheric pollution, cigarette smoke, and various materials in the environment contain certain hydrocarbons which can produce cancer. Other environmental carcinogens are alkylating agents, lactones, azo dyes and nitroso compounds (Richards, 1972).[3]

PHYSICAL AGENTS. Radiation—Studies have shown that irradiation of cells by X-rays, ultraviolet light, and other physical sources are carcinogenic (Richards, 1972). Radioactive isotopes deposited in the long bones of radium dial painters may cause sarcomas. Survivors of the Nagasaki and Hiroshima atomic blasts show an increased incidence of leukemia. A single X-ray film of the abdomen of a pregnant woman may increase the incidence of cancer, including leukemia, in the child (Richards, 1972).[3]

Viruses—For many years, it was believed that viral tumors occurred only in birds, especially chickens; later it was demonstrated that a mammalian tumor could be caused by a virus (Richards, 1972). Recent research (cf. Morton et al, 1972) suggests that there are a number of virus-like particles which are associated with various human tumors. While the origin of some of these particles is uncertain, a few known human viruses have been observed to induce cancers in lower animals. However, it has not been demonstrated conclusively that the same virus can cause tumors in man. Nevertheless, the majority of studies show that the virus materials have an oncogenic potential. While immunological and biochemical studies generally support the suggestion that some of the human viruses could be causally related to the human tumors in which they can be found, additional evidence is essential before either an etiological or purely casual role can be assigned to any of these viruses. Viruses are now regarded not only as particles that will kill cells as they multiply within those cells, but as specific particles of new genetic material which, once introduced into the cell, may initiate cancer (Watson, 1970).

GEOGRAPHIC FACTORS. Cancer of the stomach may be linked to nutritional factors which vary with geography. The Japanese, in their country, have a high incidence of stomach cancer, but show a diminished risk after emigrating to the United States. Cancer of the colon is most frequent in English-speaking countries; moreover, countries which have a high incidence of cancer of the colon show low incidence of stomach cancer. Oral cancer is rare in the United States, but prevalent in India (up to 70% of all cancers) where chewing betel nuts is customary. Esophageal cancer, generally prevalent in lower socio-economic groups, is rare in Europe and the Americas, frequent in Japan and in the Bantu region of South Africa, and common in Swedish women. Leukemia is frequent in Israel, Denmark, Japan, and the United States. Women of Chile have the highest general cancer rate in the world. They have more cancer of the uterus and stomach than any other women, but also show the lowest rate of skin, colon, and rectum cancer, as well as leukemia (Glemser, 1969).

SPECIFIC TRAUMA. Trauma is a form of irritation. It seems likely that trauma is probably a *promoting* agent, stimulating a latent neoplasm to reach a critical size (Richards, 1972). In an inveterate pipe smoker, cancer of the lip tends to develop at the place where he holds his pipe (Selye, 1956). Sexually active women show a higher incidence of cervical cancer which is rare among nuns and virgins (Selye, 1956).

GENERALIZED TRAUMA. General stress tends to *suppress* cancerous growth (Selye, 1956). Various types of clinical and experimental cancer often are significantly retarded by infections (Watanabe, 1966), intoxications and various drugs which cause much nonspecific damage. For example, it has been reported that tumors commonly retract after patients are injected with a live-bacteria tuberculosis vaccine called BCG. It also has been possible to inhibit the growth of certain tumors with large doses of anti-inflammatory hormones (e.g., ACTH); these hormones normally are secreted in large amounts during times of stress (Selye, 1956).

ISOLATION. Carcinogenesis also seems to be modified by depriving neural and non-neural structures of information. Andervont

(1941, 1944) and Muhlbock (1951) observed that mice develop spontaneous mammary tumors significantly earlier if the animals are raised in
isolation. Sanford et al (1950), who found that malignant changes can
occur in cultured cells which received no specific treatment, concluded, "apparently it is in some way the result of isolation in the
tissue-culture situation." Shelton and her colleagues (1963) demonstrated that untreated normal cells underwent malignant conversion in
a completely isologous biological environment.

Biological-Structural Variables

PHYLOGENY. Many investigators believe that it is questionable
whether the lumps and cellular accumulations found in many plants
and invertebrates have features that are associated with the malignant
tumors of mammals and other vertebrates (Good and Finstad, 1969;
Sparks, 1972). Apparently, the probability of carcinogenesis increases
with phylogenetic development. Every type of cancer affecting man
can also be found in other vertebrates but different kinds of cancer
occur in different proportions in each species, and each has its own
particular spectrum of tumors (Glemser, 1969).

ONTOGENY. Cancer appears, by and large, in the post-reproductive period of life. The majority of patients who die of cancer are
between the ages of forty-five and sixty-five. Among adults, cancers
of the breast, lungs, stomach, colon and cervix are the most common.
Childhood cancer accounts for one out of twenty-eight deaths compared to adult figures of one out of six. Cancer kills more children
between the ages of three and fourteen than any other disease.
Leukemia accounts for about one-half of these deaths (American
Cancer Society, 1975).

GENETIC BACKGROUND. Some cancers are clearly hereditary.
Among these are a cancer of the eye in children, an intestinal cancer
derived from intestinal polyposis, and some tumors of the nerve cells.
However, direct inheritance of *most* forms of cancer seems unlikely as
research on identical twins points out. Von Verschuer (1968) showed
that only 34 of 196 identical twins developed cancer more or less
simultaneously. Jarvik and Falek (1968) found that in only three cases
of sixty had twins who were hereditarily similar both contracted
cancer. In addition, if most forms of cancer were inherited, then
tumors in organs that are identically determined by heredity should be
quite common. Cases in which cancer of both kidneys, lungs, or sexual
glands have been found are medical rarities; for example, in breast
cancer, only one breast is affected in 97% of all cases.

It is clear, however, that hereditary influences exist which
predispose some individuals to cancer. Thus, an excessive aggregation
of cancer in some families is now recognized. The cancer may be of a
single site, as in a Boston family in which seven women had ovarian
cancer (Li et al, 1970). Familial cancer syndromes include ones

characterized by soft-tissue sarcomas in the children, and breast cancer in the mother, and other female relatives (Anderson, 1974; Li and Fraumeni, 1969a; Li and Fraumeni, 1969b).

GENDER.   Cancer of the colon is more common among women than among men, while cancer of the rectum is more common in males.   Lung cancer may be sex related.   Female rates from lung cancer are lower than the rate for men (American Cancer Society, 1975), although the incidence in females has been increasing as they increase cigarette smoking.   Gardner (1953) and Kaplan et al (1954) observed that lymphoid leukemia occurs less frequently and later in males.   They attributed the differential susceptibility to sex hormones; estrogens promote leukemia, whereas testosterone inhibits the disease, and castration often stimulates leukemia in males and decreases it in females.

HORMONES.   It has been established that certain cancers are hormone dependent or hormone sensitive.   Huggins (1965) obtained remissions of cancer of the prostate in men by removal of the testicles, the main source of male sex hormones controlling the activity and growth of the prostate gland.   He showed that remissions in prostatic cancer could be obtained by administering synthetic estrogens.   Breast cancer in women can be influenced by the administration of male sex hormones or by surgical removal of the ovaries which terminates female sex hormone production (Richards, 1972).

HEMOSTATIC CORRELATES.   Different types of human tumors exhibit procoagulant or fibrinolytic activity far greater than that of comparable normal cells (cf.   Gralnick, 1981).   It is clear that the coagulation system may play an important role in malignant tumors by potentiating metastases or by forming a protective environment to exclude chemotherapy from reaching the tumor.   Recent studies have suggested that the use of anticoagulation or antiplatelet drugs in certain types of tumors in conjunction with chemotherapy have resulted in clinical improvement.

Malignant disease is associated with a high incidence of vascular thrombosis or disseminated intravascular coagulation (DIC).   Coagulation disorders are most commonly observed in carcinomas, but may be seen in any type of cancer.   Patients with cancer are at high risk for thrombosis or DIC when exposed to various stimuli affecting the hemostatic system.   Other abnormalities such as shortening of whole blood clotting time and elevated levels of one or more clotting factors have been reported in malignant disease without clinically evident coagulation disorders (cf. Donati, Davidson, and Garattini, 1981).

Structural-Environment Interaction Variables

RACIAL AND ETHNIC.   Cancers of the colon and rectum are more prevalent in Jewish people and less prevalent in Japanese, Poles,

Finns, and Russians. Cancer of the prostate is more frequent among blacks than whites (Richards, 1972). Whites develop cancer of the skin more often than blacks (Urbach et al, 1972).

PERSONALITY. There are many reports in the psychiatric-psychological literature that correlations exist between personality variables and the occurrence of malignancies (Brown, 1965; Coppen and Metcalfe, 1963; Hagnell, 1965; Kissen and Eysenck, 1962). While there are many problems in interpretation due to methodological problems in most studies, there is the suggestion that cancer patients show a tendency to abnormal emotional expressiveness, either excessive control or extreme lability (Marcus, 1976) relative to normal controls and other patient groups.

Limitations of the Major Hypotheses of Carcinogenesis

Many hypotheses of carcinogenesis have been formulated during the past century. The majority emanated from the pre-experimental era (prior to 1940); carcinogenesis was ascribed to chronic irritation (Ewing, 1940), embryonal persistence (Cohnheim, 1889; Warburg, 1956), respiratory impairment (Bauer, 1963), and somatic cell mutation (Berenblum, 1974).

In an excellent review, Berenblum (1974) points out that five lines of general criticism may be leveled against the various early hypotheses: confusion between cause and effect; inadequacy of appropriate techniques for testing the hypotheses; oversimplification of the nature of neoplasia with overemphasis on increased growth rate; and confining attention to certain types of neoplasia only, and then generalizing from the particular.

Modern speculation is restricted to a few inter-related hypotheses, e.g. carcinogenesis as caused by viruses (Freeman et al, 1971; Huebner et al, 1972; Watson, 1970), protein deletion (Heidelberger and Moldenhauer, 1956; Jacob and Monod, 1961; Miller, 1970; Miller and Miller, 1953; Pitot and Heidelberger, 1963; Ross, 1953) and immunological deficiency (Burnet, 1968; Good and Finstad, 1969; Levey and Medawar, 1966; Miller, 1961; Prehn, 1971). Contemporary hypotheses are all based on genetic principles, the hypotheses differing from one another according to whether the postulated change is in the DNA code of the cell, at the RNA transcription or translation level, or in the gene control system, with the immunological hypothesis allowing for all of the above (cf. Berenblum, 1974). The impetus for a genetic basis of carcinogenesis stems from the fact that an essential attribute of a neoplasm is its irreversibility after the second stage (promotion) has obtained, i.e., the handing on of newly-acquired information to subsequent generations of daughter cells after repeated cell division.

Each of the contemporary hypotheses has specific strengths and weaknesses (cf. Berenblum, 1974), and each is adequate to partially explain general cancer phenomena; but no single hypothesis provides an approach capable of handling within its theoretical framework the broad range of variables known to be associated with carcinogenesis. Further, each hypothesis has significant limitations vis-à-vis conceptualization of the generally assumed basic unity of all forms of carcinogenesis.

Basic Principles of Carcinogenesis

Berenblum (1974: 289-291) has compiled a number of basic considerations which any hypothesis of tumor causation must address if it is to be acceptable even as a preliminary working hypothesis of carcinogenesis.

1. The primary step in neoplastic transformation is a local phenomenon, presumably affecting a single cell. The resulting tumor mass thus represents a clone, a strain of cells descending in culture from a single cell. Since the newly acquired neoplastic properties are transmitted to daughter cells on cell division, the neoplastic change is, in effect, an irreversible process (this does not necessarily conflict with the rare occurrence of tumor regression, which probably represents a reversal to a dormant state as far as the tumor cells dying and/or being eliminated).

2. Every kind of cell in the body is potentially capable of undergoing neoplastic transformation, thus giving rise to the many different kinds of tumors. Each kind of tumor breeds true to type (though progressive anaplasia may occur after repeated transplantation). This structural and functional specificity also applies to the various tumor types according to their tissues of origin. Each tumor displays its own morphology and behavior pattern.

3. Carcinogenesis is a multi-step process. Apart from the initiation-promotion process previously described, there are further post-carcinogenic changes of an irreversible nature that can occur in the life of a tumor (Foulds, 1954) such as the transformation of a benign into a malignant tumor; the loss of hormonal dependency in a tumor which was initially hormone-dependent; loss of responsiveness to certain chemotherapeutic agents to which the tumor was initially responsive; the possibility of a specific oncogenic virus eventually disappearing from a virus-induced tumor, etc. (Berenblum, 1974).

4. Neoplastic transformation is a rare phenomenon when considered in relation to the number of cells at risk to carcinogenic action. Although carcinogenesis is generally construed as a very common process, this is only true with respect to the number of persons (or animals) affected per total of the population.

Moreover, a comprehensive model of carcinogenesis must be able to take into account multiplicity of inciting agents (including inciting-agent lack), the possibility of true spontaneous tumor development, and the broad range of environmental and biological variables known to influence carcinogenesis. Finally, a working model of carcinogenesis should provide a theoretical framework in which the assumed basic unity of all forms of carcinogenesis may be conceptualized.

THE HOLISTIC APPROACH TO CARCINOGENESIS

Recent findings and conceptual developments (cf. Petrinovich, 1979) in the sciences, coupled with the foregoing review of an increasingly broad array of variables known to be associated with carcinogenesis, suggest the need for a new conceptual approach or paradigm in the study of carcinogenesis. The dualistic metaphysics of the vitalistic and mechanistic paradigms have been hopelessly outdated by the findings of contemporary physics. At the macrolevel, for example, relativity theory has demonstrated the incontrovertibility of matter and energy. At the microlevel, quantum mechanics has shown that matter exists neither as a particle or a wave but rather as a "field" which manifests different forms depending on the conditions under which it is observed (Battista, 1977).

In the realm of epistemology, relativity theory points out that the objective stance of the mechanistic paradigm is illusory and inadequate. It suggests e.g., that two observers traveling at different velocities near the speed of light may observe the same event occurring at different times and differing in length and mass. Studies in quantum mechanics point out that a certain amount of negentropy (information) is necessary to conduct an observation and that these observations not only alter and determine what we are observing but also make it impossible to measure all of its characteristics simultaneously (Heisenberg's uncertainty principle). Thus a perspectivistic or a relativistic epistemology is indicated (Battista, 1977).

As is generally recognized, the mechanistic paradigm supplanted the vitalistic paradigm in the nineteenth century because of the capacity of deterministic causality to more fully account for phenomena such as breathing and the circulation of blood, phenomena which up to that time had been explained as the direct manifestation of a vitalistic force (Battista, 1977). The vitalist's last stronghold for some time had been the mechanist's inability to explain the apparent purposiveness of organisms. One of the strengths of the holistic paradigm is its ability to account for purposive behavior without positing more than one kind of force. This is accomplished by viewing all interactions to occur as information processing loops or servomechanisms (Miller, Galanter, and Pribram, 1960). The result has been a better understanding of such phenomena as drinking, eating, mating, and thinking, and the development of purposive machines such as thermostats, self-guiding missiles and computers. In addition, the probabilistic causality of the holistic paradigm has been shown to be more consistent with the findings of quantum mechanics than is the deterministic causality of the mechanistic paradigm (Battista, 1977).

Finally, the social and behavioral sciences have found the mechanistic paradigm untenable because its reductionistic mode of analysis and entropic kinetics cannot handle the phenomena of novelty and/or the emergence of higher forms of complexity. The vitalistic position that ontogenesis and phylogenesis are the inherent properties of a vitalistic or spiritual force does nothing to explain the emergence of form and discourages further investigation. The open system kinetics of the holistic paradigm makes it possible to understand and model the process of development without pointing to any new forces and without contradicting the second law of thermodynamics (Battista 1977).

Kuhn (1962) has pointed out that paradigmatic shifts tend to occur rapidly and simultaneously in all fields of science. The Copernican revolution represented a shift from a vitalistic to a mechanistic framework. The mechanistic paradigm dominated in the nineteenth century, and it culminated in the development of Newtonian physics which was thought to reveal the fundamental laws of the universe. Today contemporary scientific findings and theoretical developments have rendered classical physics and the mechanistic tradition untenable.   The old concepts of energy, force and causality are being replaced by the newer concepts of probability, information and organization in all fields of science (Battista, 1977).

These considerations lead to the conclusion that a holistic paradigm is better suited to serve as a guiding conceptual framework for understanding cancer, as well as health and disease broadly considered. The next chapter will describe some basic premises of a holistic approach to the problem of carcinogenesis. The approach appears to be capable of providing a greater *synthesis* of data on carcinogenesis than has been possible before. It draws heavily from and builds upon knowledge emerging from the study of control systems (von Bertalanffy, 1950; Miller, 1973) and on recent advances in cognitive-developmental psychophysiology, and neuropsychology.

Chapter 2 The Underlying Premises of the Developmental-Structural Approach: The Concepts of Cognitive Structure, Information, Optimal Information Load, and Homeostasis

> Nasrudin is out riding when he sees a group of horsemen. Thinking that this may be a band of robbers, Nasrudin gallops off hastily. The other men, who are actually friends of his, say, "I wonder where Nasrudin is going in such a hurry?" and trail after him to find out. Nasrudin, feeling himself pursued, races to a graveyard, leaps the fence, and hides behind a tombstone. His friends arrive and, sitting on their horses, lean over the wall to ask, "Why are you hiding behind that tombstone, Nasrudin?"
>
> "It's more complicated than you realize," says Nasrudin, "I'm here because of you, and you're here because of me."
>
> Old Sufi Joke

THE CONCEPT OF COGNITIVE STRUCTURE

Premise 1: Prior experience (including phylogenetic "experience") is represented somatically by structures (including physiological and "psychological" structures) which are built up and which, in turn, actively organize subsequent experience(s) in related contexts (Furst, 1971; Ornstein, 1972).

Throughout much of the last few centuries, behavioral scientists and philosophers have generally assumed that all animal behavior (including human) is learned through adaptive experience in the environment. Evidence from ethological studies, however, points out that while some behaviors are ontogenetically learned, (i.e., through experience after individual birth), some are innate (i.e., have developed through phylogenetic experience) and most are a gradual accommodation of genetic instructions to the specific features of the animal's environment (cf. Hanna, 1970).

There is abundant support for the notion of phylogenetically inherited behavior and perception patterns (Hanna, 1970). One example is K. Hoffman's discovery of a kind of computing mechanism in the starling which enables him to guide himself by deducing the point of the compass from the sun—when this same starling has not, up until that time, been allowed to see the sun: or the way in which a male satticid spider, reared in total ignorance of the larger, more ferocious female, already "knows" that she is of his species and exactly the kind of movements he must make in his courting dance or be devoured by the female. Although ontogenetically unlearned, he makes no mistake.

These and a host of other ethological studies (cf. Hanna, 1970) make it clear that no animal comes into this world as a *tabula rasa* waiting for ontogenetic experience to inscribe its lessons. Indeed, no neonate animal is "new;" he is, rather, infinitely old with a continuous history as long as biological time itself. Every newborn animal, every man, is already armed with a somatic wisdom encoded neurophysiologically in its body. Hanna (1970: 99-100) writes:

> And thus all species of animals bear within them a structured past, and they are currently adapting their structures of behavior (and perception) to the particular present environment; and thus, are also genetically transferring these past and present structures into the generations of the future, who, themselves, will continue the same process.

The cerebral cortex of the brain, a six-layered mantle of cells covering the cerebrum, is the most recent neural system to develop in the course of evolution. Fish have no cerebral cortex, amphibians have only a rudimentary one, and reptiles and birds have a small and poorly developed cortex. The more primitive mammals have a relatively small, smooth cortex. As the phylogenetic scale is ascended, the amount of cortex relative to the total amount of brain tissue increases in a regular manner. Within primates, this same relationship is observed: more primitive monkeys, such as the squirrel monkey and marmoset, have relatively small fissureless cortical surfaces. More advanced primates, such as the rhesus monkey, chimpanzee and man, have enormous and disproportionate increases in amount of cerebral cortex. Generally, there is a correlation between the extent of cortical development for a species, its phylogenetic position, and the degree of complexity and modifiability characteristic of its behavior (Thompson, 1967).

The cerebral cortex, particularly the frontal areas, continues to be built up with ontogenetic experience. In turn, this physiological structure actively organizes subsequent experience in related contexts. Increased ontogenetic experience is associated with the building up of cortical expectancies or models of stimulus configurations and contingencies, as well as the building up of plans for acquiring and evaluating information and for performing certain behaviors. That is, experience builds up properties in the brain which serve to make order out of incoming sensory information. These properties will be referred to as cognitive structure. The term is used here in the sense used by writers including Piaget (1952, schema), Lawrence (1963, coding response), Miller, Galanter and Pribram (1960, plans), Neisser (1967, constructions), and Furst (1970, perceptual automatizations). These acquired structures choose which inputs of stimulus configurations and contingencies to process at a relatively high rate, and which at a relatively low rate (i.e., to filter). Cognitive (cortical) structure converts the environmental situation per se into stimuli, occasions for action or emotion, to which the organism responds in terms of "meaning."

According to Neisser (1967), these structures, when activated, constitute the organism's experience, perception being regarded as an active constructive or synthetic process. In this view, structures need not be simple sensory analyzers, such as one which signals the occurrence of a simple attribute like "green," nor do they need to be experientially concrete, such as a specific memory structure representing the face of a friend. The facts of cognition and memory argue for the proposition that structures might be very abstract or schematic. Such schemas, which play a large part in the theories of cognitive psychologists (Bartlett, 1932; Piaget, 1952), would be used by a person as a guide or rough outline for constructing an experience or a memory of some event with internally-provided content. According to Furst (1970), schemas suggest the operation of some high-level program which integrates subprograms and is more suggestive of a process than are unitary "trace" ideas.

Accordingly, the concept of attention deals mainly with the selection of cognitive structures appropriate to the situation. An organism thrown into a novel situation will try to make sense out of it; he will succeed to the extent that he can relate the sensory information to existing cognitive structures—or rather, to the extent to which he can activate a well-integrated set of structures which models (matches) the sensory input. If the organism is unsuccessful, he can still make sense of it by creating new, well-integrated schemata or cognitive models. When this need arises, a state of novelty or uncertainty is said to exist which calls forth the activation of many previously unrelated bits and pieces of cognitive structure in an attempt to synthesize a new structure and thus reduce the uncertainty. If this process is successful, the result is the establishment of stable and well-integrated schemata which are adequate for the situation in that they provide good models into which incoming sensory data get broken down. Thus an organism, involved in creating new structures (models), is sampling *sensory* information at a high rate because the lack of cognitive structure results in inefficiency in gathering the sensory data needed for the immediate perceptual task, and because the organism must construct models of the environment which include as much information as possible in order to optimize his chances of survival in the environment. One might say that such an organism is paying more attention to the sensory environment, or is even more conscious of it than an organism which is merely monitoring the environment to insure continuing goodness-of-fit of his schemata and extracting the pieces of sensory information which the internal model defines as relevant (Furst, 1971).

Consider the information an adult processes from a "desk" relative to a child's processing of the same desk. The child, not having much previous experience with desks, would notice qualities which the adult might ignore, such as the highly polished oak desk-top, or perhaps the tarnished color of the often-used drawer handles; i.e., the sensory qualities of the stimulus configuration. The adult, on the other hand, probably would attend more to the *conceptual-ideational* qualities of the desk; i.e., his attention would be directed by certain tests associated in his experience with desks. These tests might take the form of internal questions such as: Does the object have a horizontal writing surface at some optimal distance from the floor? Is the horizontal writing surface supported in some way to insure stability? Having identified the stimulus configuration as a desk with these questions, he might ask further questions about its utility for him: whether the desk contains drawers, or whether there is ample space for a typewriter, etc. There is a phenomenological difference between one's first perception of a stimulus configuration relative to subsequent perceptions of the same stimulus. (These differences are discussed in more detail in Premises 3 and 5.)

There is much experimental evidence that the brain actively structures its own input. It has been demonstrated that the cerebral cortex (particularly the so-called association areas of the cortex) is not merely the passive recipient of incoming sensory stimulation, but rather exerts an active controlling influence at many levels of sensory input (Dewson et al, 1966; Spinelli and Pribram, 1966; Spinelli and Pribram, 1967). For example, Pribram and his colleagues have demonstrated corticofugal (efferent) influences as far peripherally as the cochlear nucleus and the optic tract. Changes in click- and flash-evoked recovery cycles were shown in these locations; even the size and occasionally the shape of receptive fields of units in the visual system could be altered by stimulation of the association areas of the cortex.

THE CONCEPT OF INFORMATION

Premise 2: Central nervous system structures process information from stimulus events and configurations.

"Information" is used in the current mathematical sense of the term first suggested by Hartley (1928) and later developed by Shannon (1948). Historically, the development of information theory received its main impetus from the needs of electrical engineers working on communication problems, the goal of which was to design, in the most efficient manner possible, a system which would transmit any message that might arise. The focus here is on the *capacity* to transmit information or on what might be called potential information. The word information in communication theory relates not so much to "what you do say," as to "what you could say." Information refers to the degrees of freedom (i.e., lack of constraint) that exist in a given situation to choose among signals, symbols, messages or patterns to be transmitted (von Neumann, 1958). Shannon (1948) was the first to suggest a way of calculating this capacity. He suggested that entropy (a measure of the degree of randomness of a system) is the measure of this capacity[4] and he developed the specific functional form of this measure.[5]

Potential information is vital to communication. Without the element of potential variety and uncertainty about what will come next, there is no information transmission. Cherry (1957) uses the illustration of a bookbinder's error that made every page of a book the same. Since the pages are all alike, only the first page has the potential to convey information. He states, "to set up communication, the signals must have at least some surprise value, some degree of unexpectedness, or it is a waste of time to transmit them." Thus it would appear that potential information varies directly with the entropy, so that high entropy (disorganization, randomness, unexpectedness, etc.) implies high potential information.

However, as Gatlin (1972) points out, one cannot conclude that as the entropy increases, the information always increases; rather, there is a "dimensionality" to information. She writes (Gatlin, 1972: 49):

> We cannot simply equate high entropy with high information as the communications engineer has done. Let us take a simple example. A library obviously contains stored information. The information is stored in a linear sequence of symbols ordered according to the constraints of a language. The sequences are organized into books and periodicals, and these are carefully ordered on shelves and neatly catalogued. Everywhere order and constraint are associated with the information storage process. This is a state of lowered entropy. If we were to take each page of each book, cut it into single-letter pieces and mix them in one jumbled heap, the entropy would unquestionably increase, but the stored information would decrease. Stored information, the "what we do say" of Weaver's statement, is associated with the ordering process brought about by the constraints of a language or any organized information storage process. Since stored information varies inversely with entropy, lowered entropy means a higher capacity to store information.

The implication of these notions for transmission of potential information (information flow) in a biological structure capable of information storage is obvious. Studies on the "orienting response" suggest that information flow in a given CNS structure (cortex, geniculate body, etc.) varies directly with the degree of mismatch between an expected stimulus configuration and/or event contingency and the perceived stimulus configuration; i.e., with the degree of novelty or "surprisingness" obtaining in the structure-environment interaction. A mismatch produces a generalized "orienting reaction" (Sokolov, 1960) accompanied by an increase in the level of physiological activation in the structure relative to the pre-novel stimulus baseline. With repeated exposure to a stimulus configuration and/or event contingency and accompanying "information storage," the structure forms a mental model which "predicts" the stimulus configuration and/or event contingencies; "habituation" occurs, the mismatch is resolved, information flow decreases, and physiological activation returns to baseline levels. The suggestion is important for developmental (experiential) considerations since information storage varies with development and experience in influencing potential information or information flow.

Premise 3: Information varies in quantity and in reference.

The brain processes varying *amounts* of information (e.g., bits per second) and information may be garnered from the sensory components of stimulus configurations (e.g., intensity, magnitude, color) and/or from the cognitive-ideational attributes of the same stimulus configurations (e.g., configuration, quality, quantity). The distinction between sensory and cognitive-ideational information is highlighted in Furst's (Furst, 1970) discussion of phenomenological differences between first and later perceptions of stimulus configurations. In Furst's example, a newly purchased camera has just arrived through the mail, an event which has been anticipated for several weeks. On seeing the camera for the first time, Furst suggests that it is likely that one would attend first to primarily the sensorial quality of the device, i.e., the contrast of the black textured vinyl against smooth brushed aluminum, or perhaps the subtle color of the coating of the fine optical glass. Several weeks later, while one is still cognizant of all the physical (sensory) characteristics of the camera, in the sense that he could tell a questioner about their presence or absence, he does not "notice" them as he picks up the camera to take pictures with it. He is still conscious or aware of the camera, but at a more ideational or cognitive level than before.

Premise 4: The brain has a limit as to the rate of information it can accept.

A limited channel capacity has been aptly demonstrated by experiments on absolute judgements in perception and in memory (Miller, 1956), dichotic listening (Broadbent, 1965), and shadowing

(Cherry, 1957). Recent renewal of interest among psychologists in topics dealing with the old mentalistic construction of "attention" attests to consequences of this limit (Furst, 1970). Thus, to be attentive to one item or event in the environment is to be less attentive to another; similarly, when an organism attends to some internal model of a given stimulus or environment in the form of a memory of an event or things, it has less available channel capacity for processing the sensory information associated with the same event or thing, and vice versa (Ornstein, 1972).

Premise 5: The amount of sensory information processed from a given environmental stimulus configuration and/or stimulus event contingency is generally synonymous with the level/amount of physiological activation in the central nervous system (CNS).

Presentation of a novel or unexpected stimulus produces a generalized orienting reaction (Sokolov, 1960). This orienting response is accompanied by an increase in the level of CNS activation relative to the pre-novel stimulus baseline. The purpose of the physiological changes, in general terms, is to make the individual more sensitive to incoming sensory stimuli so that he is better equipped to discern what is happening and to mobilize the body for whatever action may be necessary. With repeated exposure, the organism forms a neural or mental model which predicts the stimulus object configurations and/or stimulus event contingencies, and habituation occurs, during which physiological activation returns to baseline levels. There also occurs an accompanying decrease in the perceived sensory impressiveness of the stimulus object or events (e.g., as described in Premise 3 in the example of the newly purchased camera).

The concomitance of enhanced sensory experience and increased amounts and/or levels of physiological activation relative to the normal human adult state is well-known in various altered states of consciousness, including REM sleep, waking childhood experience, psychotomimetic drug trips, and certain lower mammal states (cf. de la Peña, 1971; Steinschneider et al, 1966; Weale, 1961). Duffy (1962) has also reviewed a broad range of studies and concludes that, excluding very high levels of sensory stimulation, sensory sensitivity increases with physiological activation.

Thus, information processing obtaining during a given state of consciousness in a given environmental situation is a function of the extent of mismatch between the stimulus configuration and the organism's expectancies of the stimulus configuration and is generally synonymous with the level of physiological activation in the CNS. The amount of arousal, or activation, or amount of sensory information processing is not conceived as some quantitative change in intensity or in the energy level in the CNS, but as a change in the *uncertainty* (and thus the information) of the CNS. Thus, the low-voltage, mixed-frequency pattern in the EEG which obtains during the orienting response to novelty in the waking environment connotes an activation pattern. This pattern is called desynchronization because it presumably reflects the cessation of synchronous firing of a large population of single units; it is an activation pattern because it signifies a decrease in redundancy of information carried by the population of cells (Pribram, 1967).

THE CONCEPTS OF OPTIMAL INFORMATION LOAD AND HOMEOSTASIS

Premise 6: The brain has an optimal range of sensory information flow for organized perceptual-cognitive-behavioral function and for feelings of relaxation. Information flow above or below this optimal range effects a disorganization of waking perceptual-cognitive-behavioral function and the experience of "anxiety" (Ashby, 1963; Berlyne, 1960; Hebb, 1955; Miller, 1960).

Studies of sensory deprivation have shown that the relative absence or diminution of sensory stimulation produces hallucinations, paranoid delusions, bewilderment, hyperactivity, anxiety and impaired mental functioning in the human adult brain (Smith et al, 1967; Zuckerman, 1969).   By the same token, the input of too much disorganized, patternless, chaotic, sensory stimulation often seems to have similar effects (Ludwig, 1971; Ludwig, 1972).

The concept of an optimal level of stimulation or arousal has had a long history. It can be traced to its origins in the Wundt (1910) concept of the relation between affective tone (pleasant-unpleasant) and stimulus intensity, and the Yerkes-Dodson (1908) law relating "rapidity of habit formation" to "stimulus strength." However, the main thrust and refinement of the concept was developed in the 1950s, coincident with studies of sensory deprivation and the surge of interest in exploratory and stimulus-seeking behavior in infrahuman species. McClelland et al (1953) suggested that small deviations from an adaptation level of stimulation produce pleasant effects while large ones produce unpleasantness.   Leuba (1955, 1962) posited that when overall stimulation is low, reactions which increase stimulation are learned, but when overall stimulation is high, reactions which decrease stimulation are more readily learned; i.e., responses which maintain an optimal level of stimulation are favored.   Fiske and Maddi (1961) emphasized the need for variation in stimulation, and suggested that individuals exhibit reliable differences in this need.

Another group of theorists formulated the "optimal level" construct in terms of "level of physiological activation."   Hebb and Thompson (1954) postulated that organisms "act so as to produce an optimal level of excitation," excitation referring to cortical activation.   Schlosberg (1954), Hebb (1955), and Malmo (1959) used an inverted U-shaped function to describe the relation between activation and behavioral efficiency.   Berlyne (1960) stated the hypothesis as follows: "For an individual organism at a particular time, there will be an optimal influx or arousal potential. Arousal potential that deviates in either an upward or a downward direction from this optimum will be drive-inducing or aversive" (p. 194). Lindsley (1957, 1961) described feedback control mechanisms between the sensory receptors, the reticular activating system, and the cortex which control the level of incoming stimulation and thereby modulate the cortical level of activation.

Jean Hamilton (1981) has provided the most cogent graphic conceptualization to date regarding the experience of boredom, interest and/or positive affect and overexcitation. The conceptualization, with some modifications, appears in Figure 1.

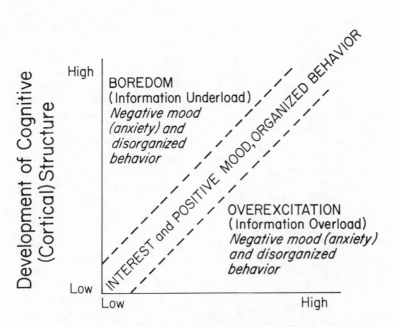

Amount of Information in Environment (External and Internal)

Figure 1

Boredom accompanied by anxiety is posited to obtain when there is a mismatch between the information provided by the environment (relatively low) and the information organizing capacity of the brain (relatively high). The experience of interest, accompanied by a positive mood and the absence of anxiety, obtains when there is a close match between information provided by the environment and the information organizing capacity of the brain. Overexcitation accompanied by anxiety occurs when there is a mismatch between environmental information (relatively high) and the information organizing capacity of the brain (relatively low). This conceptualization helps to explain the "paradoxical" observation that many individuals feel relaxed during strenuous physical activity, sports and games, risk-taking behaviors (gambling), ingestion of stimulants (alcohol, caffeine, nicotine), etc. (Davidson and Schwartz, 1976; Suebak and Stoyva, 1980). These activities apparently rectify the anxiety (boredom) associated with insufficient stimulation of cortical structures obtaining in ordinary day-to-day sensory environments (Csikszentmihalyi, 1975).

Premise 7: The brain has a variety of hierarchically organized but imperfectly coupled controls through which it may effect homeostatic changes in its own information input when information falls outside the optimal range needed for organized perceptual-cognitive-behavioral function and positive mood.[6]

It is a biological fact that the cerebral cortex of the brain is equipped to reduce the impact of *excessive* sensory stimulation, either non-specifically or selectively (Dawson, 1958; Galambos, 1955; Galin, 1965; Nobel and Dewson, 1966; Silverman, 1967). Similarly, the brain has protective mechanisms which provide "turning-on" or "augmenting," information-processing responses when the environment provides an excessively low amount of stimulation or information. The experience of sensory deprivation often precipitates hallucinations and delusions, both of which act to rectify the low level of physiological activation and/or information processing obtaining as a consequence of the information deprivation (de la Peña, 1971; Smith et al, 1967; Zuckerman, 1969). Hallucinations are associated with a very high physiological activation level in the CNS, which accompanies the endogenously-produced high rate of information processing provided the conscious brain by previously subconscious information. Delusions also seem to increase the overall information processing of the CNS, since they are associated with the individual's paying attention to environmental cues that the conscious brain might find irrelevant and hence unworthy of attention. In addition, most delusions increase the overall perceived uncertainty of the environment, and thus make the environment a bit more interesting and exciting (i.e., the deluded person may convince himself that he is the focus of a vicious plot, or the cynosure of attention, etc.).

Many of the phenomena reported by subjects in sensory deprivation studies (Zuckerman, 1964), as well as behavioral effects (Zubek, 1969), may be regarded as attempts by the brain to increase the intensity and variety of stimulation, and thereby increase the level of physiological activation in the CNS. These effects include restless bodily movement (Smith et al, 1967) and other forms of self-stimulation such as hallucinations and delusions (Zuckerman, 1969). Subjects typically talk aloud to themselves, hum and attempt to contact the experimenter on various pretexts. In attempting to sum up the sensory deprivation literature, Schultz (1965:30) suggested a homeostatic mechanism which he called "sensoristasis," a term he defined as a drive of cortical arousal which impels the organism (in the waking state) to strive to maintain an optimal level of sensory varia- tions . . . ." Sensory deprivation also has been found to increase the organism's responsivity to meaningless stimuli such as designs (Vernon and McGill, 1960), series of tones or light flashes (Jones and McGill, 1967; Jones et al, 1961) or randomly arranged color stripes (Zuckerman and Haber, 1965). Jones (1969) has summarized this body of research with the formulation of a homeostatic "information drive" interpre- tation of the results. According to Jones, information drive is homeostatic in the sense that both relatively high and relatively low levels of stimulus information induce states which motivate responses serving to maintain some intermediate level of information transmis- sion (: 206).

Thus, homeostatic "protective reactions" of the brain are best demonstrated in instances of sensory deprivation and sensory inunda- tion. Individuals in a cubicle who are provided minimum information develop alterations in consciousness. Most of these reactions (hallu- cinations, paranoid delusions, bodily hyperactivity) seemingly repre- sent an attempt by the CNS to provide an enhanced level of stimula- tion for itself. The converse, information overload, and/or extreme CNS activation, is frequently accompanied by behavioral and con- ceptual inactivity, which minimizes additional information processing (Ludwig, 1972; Silverman, 1968; Venables, 1960; Venables and Wing, 1962).

Other indirect evidence for homeostatic control of sensory input comes from studies of hyperactive children. A majority of these children, compared to normal children matched for age and socio- economic status, generally show significantly *lower* levels of physiolo- gical activation (Cohen and Douglas, 1972; Knopp et al, 1972; Satter- field and Dawson, 1971; Satterfield et al, 1972; Spring et al, 1974). Satterfield and Dawson (1971) and de la Peña (1971: Chapter 9) were the first investigators to suggest that the increased energy output, seen clinically in a majority of hyperactive children, is *secondary* to lowered levels of physiological arousal and/or sensory information processing, and probably represents an attempt by the understimulated brain to rectify its own low level of activation and/or information processing to a higher, more optimal level needed for organized cortical function.

The concept of homeostasis is at the core of this premise; at the core of homeostasis is the concept of feedback. Many excellent descriptions of feedback and self-correcting systems exist (cf. Gaar- der, 1975), so further elaboration is not required here. Suffice it to say here that the idea of circular causation and self-corrective systems was generalized at the end of World War II by Norbert Wiener and engineers working with the mathematics of non-living systems. The principle of feedback now forms the cornerstone of modern-day biology, since the self-corrective circuit and its many variants pro- vided the possibility for modeling the adaptive actions of organisms.[7]

The work of John Lacey and Peter Venables has served to

introduce the concept of "imperfect-coupling" of cortical controls in the rectification of information deficits and overload.   Prior to Lacey's work, psychophysiology had accepted the premises of unitary activation theory, which equates autonomic, behavioral, and cortical activation (information) processes, and depicts a unidimensional continuum of activation (information processing) ranging from coma to the most excited and disorganized forms of behavior (Duffy, 1962; Lindsley, 1951).   Lacey (1967), however, marshalled considerable evidence indicating that cortical, autonomic, and behavioral activation may be considered as different forms of activation; the different kinds of activation are viewed as imperfectly coupled, complexly interacting information processing systems which do not always change at the same time or in the same direction. According to Lacey (1967:21):

> Activation theory and stress theory require that correlational matrices of those physiological variables said to measure arousal exhibit sizeable communality among measures.   Many, if not most, reported matrices are disappointing: correlations among autonomic measures themselves and among autonomic and electroencephalographic variables are low, frequently approaching zero . . . the implication of idiosyncratic patterning of somatic responses for activation theory . . . [is that] . . . the degree of activation assigned to a subject or to a stressor condition may depend strikingly on the variable chosen for study.

Venables (1975), like Lacey, believes that it is no longer valid to assume a unitary dimension of activation. He urges psychophysiologists to recognize that indices of activation, which in the past have been said to measure it, have particular biological functions of their own; these functions need to be more fully understood before they can be related to more behavioral concepts.

In summary, excesses or deficits of information load are not necessarily redressed "all of a piece" (non-specifically). Excesses or deficits of sensory information, relative to some optimal range of sensory flow, can be redressed either non-specifically *or* selectively (Dawson, 1958; Galambos, 1955), at various stages of sensory input, and in a variety of waking sensory input channels (e.g., skeletal muscle, autonomic and cortical activation; behavioral activation, sleep, etc.). Which input stage(s) are and the combination of sensory input channel(s) utilized presumably depends on environmental-situational demands (i.e., the psychophysiologist's "stimulus-response specificity") and on the individual's genetic make-up ("response stereotypy").

Premise 8: One variety of sensory control processes is manifested by the tonic and phasic events of sleep.

During sleep, the adapting brain employs sensory information controls to help effect an optimal range and distribution of circadian sensory information flow that is conducive to organized waking perceptual-cognitive-behavioral function and the experience of interest-relaxation. These sleep, sensory-control processes have been extensively described in a recently published book (de la Peña, 1978), so only a conceptual skeleton is provided here.

Generally, non-Rapid Eye Movement (NREM) and Rapid Eye Movement (REM) sleep are not considered in the context of brain control theory. However, there is much evidence to suggest that both states of consiousness, and their associated phasic events, may be considered as control processes by which the brain may effect some optimal range of circadian sensory flow and activation for organized function and relaxed mood.

Non-REM Sleep as a Brain Sensory Information Control Process. With the exception of sweat gland activity (GSR),[8] NREM sleep is a time of relative CNS quiescence and regularity compared to quiet wakefulness and REM sleep. Blood pressure, respiration and heart rate show low values and little temporal and amplitude variability. A relatively low body temperature, high basal skin resistance, low urinary output and pupillary constriction are other physiological indices which differentiate NREM from REM sleep (Dement, 1969). Dream reports from NREM sleep are described as being conceptual-ideational, thought-like, more plausible, and more concerned with contemporary waking life than REM dream reports (Foulkes, 1962; Rechtschaffen et al, 1963), suggesting low amounts of sensory flow during NREM sleep. Broughton (1965, 1968) points out that dream reports of any type become less frequent with progression through stages 1 to 4 of NREM sleep, and that the occasional confusional episodes with impairment of recall occurring out of NREM sleep may not accurately reflect preceding mental activity, but possibly is an artifact of such arousals (Broughton, 1975). Generally, the amount of NREM sleep, particularly stage 4, varies directly with cumulative waking sensory flow, suggesting a homeostatic restorative function for sensory information processing channels. For example, the increased sensory flow and activation during wakefulness in the following conditions is associated with increases in slow wave sleep: exercise (Baekeland and Lasky, 1966; Browman, 1980; Horne and Porter, 1975; but Baekeland, 1970; Walker et al, 1978 contend the finding), increased visual sensory load (Horne and Walmsley, 1976; Ryback and Lewis, 1971), and the childhood state.

REM Sleep Phasic Events as a Brain Sensory Control Process. The early hypothesis (Aserinsky and Kleitman, 1953) that rapid eye movement (REM) sleep was *the* physiological correlate of remembered dreaming has gradually been replaced by a statistical viewpoint in which the REM-NREM dichotomy of sleep is thought to predict variations in the quality of the dream report: REM dream reports being, on the average, more sensorial-perceptual, vivid, active, colorful, bizarre, strange, etc., in quality; NREM reports being more plausible, conceptual-ideational, static, and more concerned with contemporary waking life (Dement, 1969; Dorus et al, 1971; Foulkes, 1962). More recent study has further suggested that the REM/NREM sleep dichotomy for predicting variations in quality of the dream, seems to reflect the relative presence or absence of phasic events (short-lived, discontinuous events such as REMs, muscle twitches, etc.) during each stage of sleep—the probability of phasic events occurring at a given time being generally higher during REM sleep (Foulkes and Pope, 1972; Molinari and Foulkes, 1969). For example, Molinari and Foulkes (1969) studied the subjective correlates of brief periods of REM bursts and of ocular quiescence with REM sleep. They interpreted REMs as a sign of overall phasic event activation and examined nonvisual, as well as visual, correlates of the presence and absence of such activation. Results indicated that REM bursts were accompanied by "primary visual experience,", i.e., visual imagery experienced in an intellectually passive fashion and unaccompanied by cognitive elaboration. Periods of ocular quiescence within stage REM either were lacking in reported visual experience or produced reports of visual imagery that was being reflected upon or reacted to in a more intellectually active manner. These findings of "sensorial", as opposed to "cognitive", dream content being associated with phasic REMs were supported in a similar study by Foulkes and Pope (1972). Another study (Berger and Oswald, 1962) found a high positive correlation between the intensity (frequency, magnitude) of phasic REMs during REM sleep and the dreamer's report, upon awakening, of behavioral activity during the dream.

Parallel physiological studies have pointed out that various measures of the REMs of REM sleep may serve as an index of the overall amount of CNS activation obtaining during REM sleep. It has been reported that bursts of REMs during REM sleep are synchronized with distinctive monophasic EEG waves called ponto-geniculate-occipital (PGO) spikes (Michel et al, 1964). According to Dement et al (1969), intense bursts of the PGO spikes are almost always associated with surges of activity in other physiological systems, e.g., muscle twitches, heart rate and blood pressure changes, REMs, etc. In agreement with this notion, studies have indicated that REM bursts within stage REM are temporarily associated with a number of autonomic and somatic physiological changes, e.g., increases in respiration rate and finger pulse responses (Spreng et al, 1968), pupillary dilation (Berlucchi et al, 1964; Berlucchi and Strata, 1965), increases in blood pressure and heart rate variability (Snyder et al, 1964), electrodermal responses (Broughton et al, 1965), and muscle twitches (Prechtl and Lenard, 1967).

Thus, studies relating the phenomenological and physiological correlates of REM bursts within REM sleep in normal human adults suggest that certain measures of phasic REMs are associated with temporal segments of dream experience in which there is an enhancement of sensory flow and activation.

The REM sleep sensory control hypothesis (de la Peña, 1971, 1973) posits that REM sleep (and associated phasic events) is one of several brain control processes which has emerged concomitantly with the development (including phylogenetic development) of cognitive (cortical) structure to help the brain achieve a survival-optimizing mode of information processing for itself during a given sleep-wakefulness temporal interval. The REM sensory control hypothesis posits that REM sleep is an auxiliary, sensory-information-control process which enhances adaptation (survival) by decreasing the "sensory information boundedness" of organisms during wakefulness. That is, with increasing development of cognitive structure, an increasingly larger proportion of the brain's total sleep-waking, *sensory* (inefficient, non-goal oriented) information processing obtains during (REM) sleep, with the result that some proportionally larger amount of survival-optimizing, *cognitive-ideational* (efficient, goal-oriented) information obtains during wakefulness. Further, during REM sleep, the brain effects homeostatic compensatory changes in its processing of endogenous, sensory information (as indexed by phasic event density, intensity, latency, etc.) according to variations in the amount of waking sensory information processing.

The result is an increase in waking behavioral-perceptual flexibility and stability since conditions of low- to moderate-degree waking sensory information underload or overload can largely be rectified by the REM sleep system, with minimal recourse to changes in waking behavior (hyperactivity, hypoactivity) or in waking perception (abnormally high or low sensory thresholds) which may be deleterious to organismic survival. On the other hand, the presence of an auxiliary, sleep sensory control system increases the organism's ability to adapt to a high degree of sensory information overload-underload, since both sleep *and* waking sensory information processing controls may be employed to rectify the conditions.

A broad range of literature (cf. de la Peña, 1971) suggests that a homeostatic relation exists between amounts of sensory flow and activation occurring across the states of wakefulness and sleep, the latter being positively indexed by measures of the organization, intensity, and density of phasic REMs during REM sleep and negatively by latency to the first REMs of REM sleep. Evidence for this generalization has been reviewed elsewhere (de la Peña, 1971, 1973) so only a brief outline of experimental support will be given here:

1. *Sensory information underload-overload.* REM sleep phasic event density and intensity increase following waking sensory underload and decrease following sensory enrichment (de la Peña and Ornitz, 1973; Potter and Heron, 1972; Prevost et al, 1974; Prevost et al, 1975);

2. *Waking stress studies.* Illnesses such as colds, the flu, etc., are accompanied by lower REM intensities and densities. Individuals spending their first night in the sleep lab show lower densities and intensities of phasic REMs. This may occur because the individual is

experiencing an enhanced amount of sensory flow and activation the first night relative to subsequent nights after he has developed cognitive structure and processes a lower amount of sensory information from the same environment. Organismic-environmental interaction patterns evocative of anxiety (i.e., feelings of uncertainty, unpredictability) are often reported to be associated with decreased REM intensity and density.

3. *Phylogeny.*   Since cognitive structure is less developed at lower phylogenetic levels, the REM sleep sensory control hypothesis predicts lower amounts of REM sleep because there is relatively more sensory information processing during wakefulness.   Although there is no comparative data on phasic event intensity-density as a function of phylogenetic development, Berger (1969) has reported a generally increasing REM percentage with increasing levels of morphological complexity of organisms, especially if the percentage of total sleep spent in REM sleep is divided by the percentage of the day spent asleep for each species in order to compensate for differences in daily sleep time.

4. *Ontogeny.*   One of the most striking properties of REM sleep is its radical change with age. The percentage of total sleep spent in REM sleep drops from over 50% in infancy to less than 14% in old age (Feinberg, 1969; Roffwarg, 1966). However, REM sleep *phasic* event intensity and organization *increases* with age until young adulthood, thereafter declining. Thus, Ornitz and colleagues (Ornitz et al, 1971; Tanquay et al, 1976) report an increasing percentage of REM sleep during which eye movement bursts occur with increasing age. Prechtl and Lenard (1967) claimed that burst patterns of REMs do not occur in human neonates. Petre-Quadens (Petre-Quadens and De Lee, 1970; Petre-Quadens et al, 1971) reported results in partial agreement; although no (or very few) bursts were found for neonates in the early part of the sleep cycle during the night, a larger number were found in the later part of the sleep cycle, whereas they were found to exist in older children from the very first REM period.   According to the developmental-psychophysiological theoretical framework and REM sleep sensory control theory, children show lowered sensory flow and activation during REM sleep (as indexed by measures of phasic REM organization and intensity) because they experience enhanced sensory flow and activation during wakefulness relative to more experienced adults.

Chapter 3 The Underlying Premises of the Developmental-Structural Approach: The Concepts of Automatization, System, and Emergence

The Gods were bored so they created man. Adam was bored because he was alone and Eve was created. . . . Adam was bored alone, then Adam and Eve were bored together; then Adam and Eve and Cain and Abel were bored en famille; then the population of the world increased and the people were bored en masse. To divert themselves, they conceived the idea of constructing a tower high enough to reach the heavens. This idea itself is as boring as the tower was high, and constitutes a terrible proof of how boredom had gained the upper hand.

Soren Kierkegaard
"The Rotation Method"

THE CONCEPT OF AUTOMATIZATION

Premise 9: Information processing and/or attention becomes automatized with increments in experience.

The term automatization is a critical one in the exposition of this book's hypothesis. Ford (1929) studied the problem in the context of structuralist investigations of the effects of distracting stimuli, viewing "attention" and "automatization" as two links of a continuum which vary with perceptual experience. A similar term "automatism" is used in clinical neurology to denote states which occur during temporal lobe seizures, in which people perform complicated but inappropriate actions with no subsequent memory of them. In the psychoanalytical tradition, Hartmann (1939) described automatizing as an ego function which serves to increase perceptual efficiency by a conservation of "attention cathexis."

The psychologist Charles Furst has described automatization in information processing terms (1971: 65):

> People often refer to acts that have become so habitual that they are performed unconsciously, and it is not difficult to accept the proposition that motor skills, at least, can be in some sense automatized. But most skills that we learn are neither purely motor nor purely perceptual in nature, but some complicated mixture of both. When a person relates the common experience of driving a car over a familiar route automatically, it is not surprising to find that one of the things that he means is that he was unconscious not only of the movements of his arms and legs, but that he was also unconscious of the events going by his car's windows.
>
> Arguing from a functional point of view, it would seem that automatizing of a perceptual process would occur in order to increase the efficiency of all ongoing perceptual activity. So, it is reasonable that automatizing should be evidenced by a decrease in the activity of a perceptual system or by a decrease in the rate of information being processed by that system. It has been amply demonstrated that perceptual channels have limited capacity (Broadbent, 1958) so that any savings in the amount of information flow in a subsystem must result in a gain in the system's capability for processing other information simultaneously. That stimulus specific perceptual processes decrease in activity as a result of experience is well known (e.g., Sharpless and Jasper, 1956), and this phenomenon is known physiologically as habituation. Automatizing can be viewed as an efficient decrease in the sensory information necessary to construct a repeated perceptual event, and on a phenomenological level, this can be seen as implying the reduction of awareness of things one acquires as a result of past experience with them.

The most recent description of automatization within an information processing framework is Schiffrin and Schneider's (1977) two-stage theory of attention. Their studies demonstrate the qualitative difference between two modes of information processing: automatic detection and controlled search. Automatic detection (automatized information processing) is relatively well-learned in long-term memory, is demanding of attention only when a target is presented, is parallel in nature, is difficult to alter, to ignore, or to suppress once learned, and is virtually unaffected by information load. Controlled search, on the other hand, is highly demanding of attentional capacity, is usually serial in nature with a limited comparison rate, is easily established, altered, and even reversed by the subject, and is strongly dependent on load.

Furst provides some elegant descriptions of the phenomenology of automatization (1970: 82-92). They are worth quoting at length here.[9]

> After you habituate to a stimulus, it can still be recognized and acted upon in an apparently unconscious or automatic manner. This phenomenon is one aspect of a general tendency toward the unconscious execution of any activity which is performed habitually. Consider the case of a tourist approaching the Golden Gate Bridge for the first time and a commuter viewing it from the same spot, one car behind. What is the difference in their perceptions? They are both looking at the same object in their visual fields, taking mental note of it, and categorizing it, identifying it. They would both be able to tell you, for instance, that the color of the bridge is red, that it is suspended from two tall towers by a web of steel cable. Still, there is a sense in which the commuter, who has seen this bridge twice a day for the last seven years, is not as aware of the bridge. The color of the bridge is less vivid, the towers less imposing and graceful, the web of cables less intricate than when he himself had seen it for the first time.
>
> What the commuter would say about his unawareness is that he knows the route so well that he drives it "automatically." We use the term in everyday speech. It is a common observation, for example, while we are learning some new and complicated physical skill, like hitting a golf ball, that at some point in time the actions become unconscious. Where we once had to pay attention to the coordination of a thousand and one different muscles, now things seem to run off so smoothly that it seems automatic. The term "automatic" refers simply to our lack of mental effort or a lack of awareness. This metaphor is a fortunate one, in terms of what we have called the mental "economy" of attention.

Experimental evidence for this premise is abundant. The young or less experienced organism (including less phylogenetically experienced organisms, such as lower mammals) shows higher sensitivity (absolute thresholds) to minimal-intensity sensory stimulation in the major sensory modalities (Hinchcliffe, 1958; Sherman and Robilard, 1960; Collins and Stone, 1966; Haslam, 1969; Pare, 1969). The younger organism also shows an enhanced general level of cortical and autonomic activation (Steinschneider et al, 1966; cf. de la Peña, 1971), as

well as a relative retardation in habituation of a variety of physiological orienting responses to environmental stimulation (Nikitina, 1954;
Lynn, 1966; Vinogradova, 1961; McCance,1961; Richter, 1961; Gastaut
and Bert, 1960). For example, numerous studies show that young
children display lower sensory (pain) thresholds (Haslam, 1969), more
cardiac variability (Steinschneider et al, 1966), and a relative retardation of habituation of the orienting response (Lynn, 1966) compared to
adults.   There is also recent work showing that the capability of
organisms to habituate to stimuli is paralleled by the maturation of
cholinergic inhibitory system in the forebrain (Fibiger et al, 1970;
Moorcroft et al, 1971; Mabry and Campbell, 1974).   Marsh and
Thompson (1977) have reviewed studies of autonomic nervous system
in the elderly; in general, an underarousal hypothesis is supported.

Premise 10: Automatization is a central dimension in evolution. It is a
necessary condition for the development and/or acquisition of perceptual-motor and cognitive skills.   Its sequela is a lowering of the
intensity of consciousness, which is experienced as boredom and ennui.

Colin Wilson, the British existentialist thinker, has written bril-
liantly on the concept of automatization and its role in the acquisition
of skill and in the genesis of the experience of boredom and ennui. He
writes (1969, pp 30-72):

> I have invented a useful concept for dealing
> with this basic psychological problem; I call it the
> "robot." When a human being learns anything diffi-
> cult—to talk, to write, to calculate, to drive a car,
> to type, to speak a foreign language—he has to
> begin by concentrating upon the details of what he
> wishes to learn. Even when he has learned a basic
> French vocabulary, he finds it difficult to read
> French, because he is still thinking in English, and
> he has to translate each word into English. But
> gradually, the "remembering" process is passed on to
> a deeper level of his being, a kind of robot in his
> subconscious mind, and the robot can read French
> without having to translate it back into English. It
> is in every way more efficient than his conscious
> personality.
> All animals possess a robot to some extent—
> otherwise they would not be able to learn. But man
> has the most efficient robot of all. The cleverer he
> is, the more efficient the robot.   But the very
> efficiency of his robot is one of his greatest prob-
> lems. Because you will observe that the sense of
> freedom, of being vitally alive, tends to occur when
> you are doing something for the first time. The
> amateur actor gets far more excitement out of it

than the professional. The most blasé person becomes a schoolboy again if you get him to do
something at which he is totally inexperienced:
riding a horse, skiing, appearing on television. The
more intelligent a man is—the quicker he learns
things—the more quickly the activity is passed on to
his robot, and is done automatically. This is the
great disadvantage of the robot: that it not only
drives your car and talks French, but also takes the
excitement out of skiing or listening to a symphony.
The robot has taken over too many of our functions.
The consequence is that when life is peaceful, we
find it difficult to feel really alive.

In a more recent work, Wilson (1979: 524-525) continues his
analysis of automatization of attention and its consequences for the
acquisition of skill and the promotion of the experience of boredom.

The concept of the robot can also be used to
explain evolution. Evolution *is* the development of
the robot. Our hearts beat automatically. Our hair
and nails grow automatically. Our stomachs digest
food automatically. These functions have already
been automatised by the evolutionary process, so
that consciousness is free to deal with other problems. If I had to *think* about my breathing, I would
have no attention to spare for anything else.
For convenience, we can think of automatisa-
tion as a servant of will or spirit . . . . The aim is
always to give will (and eventually consciousness)
more freedom. But at a certain point in the
process, something began to go wrong. The problem
is that conscious awareness separates us from our
instincts. We began to lose the sense of why we
were doing all this, and so gave a free hand to the
greatest enemy of evolution: laziness. If I am free,
then I can choose whether to use my freedom to
conquer new ground, or merely to lie in the sun and
yawn. If I have lost all sense of urgency, and my
conscious mind can perceive no particular purpose,
then I am just as likely to choose inactivity. My
robot, the perfect valet, now becomes the chief
support of my laziness.

Premise 11: Excessive automatization of attentional processes is
associated with attempts to de-automatize consciousness. These
attempts may have maladaptive or adaptive consequences for the
individual and society.

Wilson, again, has captured the essence of this premise in the following passages from his recent book *Mysteries* (1979: 526-527):

> Our low-pressure consciousness can be held
> responsible for most of our major defects.   It
> produces a kind of nagging hunger for excitement
> that leads to all kinds of irrational behaviour. This
> is why gamblers gamble, sex maniacs commit rape,
> sadists inflict pain and masochists enjoy having it
> inflicted, and why men become alcoholics and drug
> addicts.   It also explains why we are so prone to
> outbreaks of criminality and mass destruction. Vio-
> lence and pain are preferable to boredom and frus-
> tration.
> Throughout his history, man has shown the same
> depressing tendency to escape his boredom through
> violence and destruction, and there is no reason to
> believe that the invention of nuclear weapons will
> improve his record. There is an element of absurd-
> ity in seeking out forms of crisis that will catapult
> him into a "wide-awake consciousness"; it is like
> persuading yourself to go out for a walk by setting
> the house on fire. On the other hand, man has also
> shown a long-standing tendency to recognise the
> futility of mere excitement, and to attempt to get
> to the root of the problem. This tendency is called
> religion.   When religious ascetics wore hair shirts
> and slept on bare planks, it was because they
> recognised instinctively that the problem was to *de-
> condition* themselves from over-reliance on the ro-
> bot.   They were trying to shake the mind awake
> through pain and discomfort. But even this remedy
> contains traces of the old "original sin," the reliance
> on external pressures.   Discomfort *can* shake the
> mind awake; but a sense of purpose can do it more
> positively and effectively.

Thus, the argument here is that evolution and/or development is
associated with automatization of attentional processes. Automatization makes possible the impressive array of perceptual, motoric, and
cognitive skills which emerge with increments in experience; it is at
the core of the development of "intelligence" as well as a great part of
what we label "creative" work in the arts and sciences. Much of great
science and art serves to help us escape the trivial everyday world and
allow us to enter a world of wider significance and meaning. Wilson
writes (1974, p. 42):

> It struck me then that the main problem of
> human life is easy to define. We live too close to
> the present, like a gramophone needle travelling

> over a record. We never appreciate the music as a whole because we only hear a series of individual notes . . . . I realised that all science has simply been man's attempt to get his nose off the gramophone record, to see things from a distance, to escape this perpetual tyranny of the present. He invented language and then writing to try to escape his worm's eye view of his own existence. Later still he invented art—painting, music, literature, to try to store the stuff of his living experience. It came to me with a shock that art is really an extension of science, not its opposite; science tries to store and correlate dead facts; art and literature try to store and correlate living facts.
>
> And then, the clearest insight of all: science is not man's attempt to reach "truth." He doesn't want "truth"—in the sense of mere "facts." He wants wider consciousness, freedom from this strange trap that holds our noses against the gramophone record. That is why he has always loved wine and music.

Thus, the development of increasingly comprehensive, sophisticated cortical and sub-cortical programs for processing information leaves the relatively experienced organism with a relatively low intensity of consciousness (boredom, ennui, loneliness, etc.) on exposure to ordinary external and internal environments. Consequently, the brain of the experienced individual is constantly attempting to rectify the low-level information flow (information underload) in order to maintain its own level of integrity and to realize some optimal range/rate of information flow for its own organized function. While some attempts at rectification are often successful and adaptive for the organism, (great works of art and science), other compensatory attempts are often maladaptive for the integrity of self and society (e.g., hyperactivity, violence for the sake of violence, hallucinations, and paranoid delusions). As the artist S. Steinberg (1978) has expressed it: "avoiding boredom is one of our most important purposes."

Empirical support for the notion of the adaptive consequences of compensatory de-automatization behaviors does not exist in the literature. However, there is a wealth of data to support the assertion that compensatory de-automatization behaviors may often be maladaptive for individuals.

Literature review on the psychophysiology of hyperactivity and explosive personality (to be described in Chapter 8) points out that low levels of information flow in the resting state are generally found in hyperactive children and adults with explosive personality. Since stimulant medication normalizes behavior in these populations, it is suggested that the excessively vigorous behavior is secondary to insufficient information flow and/or physiological activation, i.e., excessive automatization of attention. Hyperactive children and adults with explosive personality are also observed to fall asleep very easily in relatively unstimulating environments. Sleep, particularly non-REM sleep, is the end result of automatization of attention.

Literature review (cf. de la Peña, 1971) in the area of schizophrenia indicates that the performance of heterogeneous groups of schizophrenics tends to define the *extremes* on several basic response dimensions, including sensitivity to sensory stimulation (Fischer et al., 1968; Silverman, 1967) and in levels of physiological activation (Claridge and Hume, 1966; Lang and Buss, 1965; Venables, 1964; Depue and Fowles, 1974; Gruzulier and Venables, 1975). A growing body of data suggests that, contrary to popular clinical impression, the behaviorally hyperactive paranoid type of schizophrenic is *not* hypersensitive to minimal intensity stimulation and does not generally have an exceedingly high level of physiological activation (Depue and Fowles, 1974; Silverman, 1967; Silverman, 1968; Jurko et al., 1952). Rather, the hypoactive withdrawn and/or nonparanoid schizophrenic, who maintains a perceptually undifferentiated orientation toward his environment,[10] is the one who is hypersensitive (Silverman, 1968) and gives evidence of an extremely high level of CNS activation (Venables, 1960; Venables and Wing, 1962; Venables, 1963). These results suggest that the maintenance of a highly differentiated attentional set, one characteristic of the paranoid schizophrenic state, might act as a kind of sensory stimulus barrier which buffers the impact of sensory stimulation. According to Silverman (1967, p. 230):

> In sensory response studies of schizophrenics which are conducted with low or ordinary intensity ranges of stimulation, nonparanoid schizophrenics usually evidence hyperactivity (hypersensitivity) to input . . . . On the other hand, schizophrenics with paranoid subtype diagnoses tend not to evidence these behaviors and on certain of the procedures they evidence the opposite behaviors (hyposensitivity).

I posit that the evolution and maintenance of a highly differentiated cognitive delusional system, coupled with behavioral hyperactivity, both hallmarks of the paranoid schizophrenic state, represent attempts by the brain to effect a more optimal level/range of information processing when the environment fails to provide enough information necessary for organized cortical function. Most delusions would represent an attempt by the brain to increase the uncertainty (and thus the information) of the relatively unstimulating environment and/or to raise an abnormally low level of physiological CNS activation. The paranoid schizophrenic believes he is Napoleon, the target of a conspiracy, the focus of much stimulation and attention, etc. The hyperactive behavior seen in the majority of paranoid schizophrenics would also act to increase information flow and rectify sensory information underload.

Premise 12: High development of cognitive structure implies a susceptibility to disruption of organized waking perceptual-cognitive-behavioral function from sensory information underload and cognitive-ideational overload; low development of cognitive structure implies the converse.

Compared to the less experienced brain, the more experienced brain processes less sensory information from a given ordinary environment because much of it has been incorporated into "mental models of expected stimulation." The more experienced brain may be said to attend more to the conceptual-ideational attributes of the same stimulus environment. The relative "automatization" of perception may be conceptualized to result in a relative, functional sensory-information underload in encounters with ordinary day-to-day environments; the relatively low level of sensory flow and activation is associated phenomenologically with a low intensity of consciousness (Wilson, 1972; Wilson, 1969) and with the experience of boredom, ennui, depression, fatigue, and feelings of alienation from the environment. Compared to the less experienced brain, then, the more experienced one is predisposed to disorganized perceptual-cognitive-behavioral function from sensory information *underload* rather than from overload and from the resulting cognitive-ideational-information overload which the brain employs to help rectify the low sensory flow and activation within the optimal range/level needed for organized waking perceptual-cognitive-behavioral function and relaxed mood.

Minimal development of structure implies a high sensitivity to low-intensity sensory stimulation/information, and a concomitant susceptibility to disruption of organized function from information overload, and vice versa (Kacser, 1957; Thompson, 1968). Thompson (:84) has written:

> We have defined growth as an increment in redundancy. On this basis, we might then expect that a mature system that has grown more and therefore has more components that perform the same function should be better buffered against environmental change than an immature system .... Furthermore, if we conceptualize the young system as being less differentiated and less well organized, we must conclude that such reactivity as it does possess may have a rather low threshold and may produce a more total and global response. This would make it comparable to a highly sensitive homeostat that is capable of handling only a small range of environmental fluctuation situations, and will break down if the deviation it is called on to correct is too great.

Or again, in other words (Thompson, 1968):

> Growth is essentially an increment in redun-
> dancy of a system . . . . Any system that has more
> redundancy in it can withstand stress or "noise"
> more successfully. Language systems exemplify this
> principle. The probability of a message being com-
> municated is known to be greater if it contains some
> redundancy than if it contains none.[11]

The above premise implies that the greater the experience and/or
development of structure, the lower the sensitivity to minimal intensity sensory stimulation/information, and the higher the optimal range
of stimulation/information needed for optimal organization of functioning. It also implies a concomitant predisposition to experience
disruption of organized function (homeostasis) more from information
underload rather than information overload. In concrete terms, the
more experienced structure processes less information from a given
ordinary environment relative to the amount processed by a less
experienced/developed structure, because most of the information is
already in the structure's mental model of expected stimulation. The
more experienced/developed structure compensates for the paucity of
information by increasing its own activity level or seeking out
relatively stimulating, informationally rich stimulus environments (de
la Peña, 1971).

This premise is in agreement with Zuckerman's (1969:   430)
conclusions that young children have a lower optimal level of stimulation than older children and adolescents. He writes: "Optimal level of
stimulation . . . reaches a peak in adolescence, and declines thereafter.   Young children are prone to be frightened by unfamiliar
stimulation and seem to enjoy repetition of the familiar more than
older children or adults." Further corroboration is provided by Kish
(1966:140) who, upon review of the animal literature on exploratory
behavior, extrapolated a curvilinear relationship between exploratory
activity and increasing age. Exploratory behavior was minimal in very
young animals, he found, increasing with maturational status to some
maximal value, and then falling off with further increments in age.
Studies by Wekler (1956) and Levin and Forgays (1959) essentially
confirm the findings on child/adolescent preferred stimulation levels.
Further, there is some indication (Kish, 1968) that other aspects of
enhanced experience such as education attainment, intelligence level,
and perceptual-spatial-numerical aptitudes, are positively correlated
with a relatively high need for stimulation or preferred stimulation
level as assessed by Zuckerman's Sensation-Seeking Scale (SSS).[12]

The above considerations imply that the experienced/developed
structure is more likely to show disruption of organized function
(homeostasis), compared to the less experienced structure on exposure
to environments providing a minimal level of stimulation. Indirect
evidence for this is the personality theory which predicts differences
in the reaction to sensory deprivation (Harvey et al, 1961; Schroder et
al, 1967), in which a dimension of conceptual simplicity-complexity is

posited. Conceptually simple individuals process information in rigid, absolutist ways, whereas the complex person is flexible, integrative and subtle. The complex individual, according to Schroder, is able to process information more accurately and rapidly, and has a relatively high need to obtain and use information—rather than existing preferences or biases—in coping with problems. In three sensory deprivation studies based on this framework, complex people were shown to find sensory deprivation more unpleasant than conceptually simple subjects, and were more willing to comply with the demands of the experiment in order to receive rewarding information. Since older children, adolescents, and adults are more conceptually complex than young children, one could infer that sensory deprivation would be more unpleasant and hence possibly more cognitively/behaviorally disrupting for older children and adults than for the younger children (cf. Wilson, 1971).

THE CONCEPT OF SYSTEM

Premise 13: The foregoing premises apply not only at the CNS-organism level of analysis, but also at CNS and non-CNS sub- and supra-levels of organization in nature.

A system is defined as a complex of components in interaction (von Bertalanffy, 1967). General system theory attempts to discern those principles that apply to systems in general, irrespective of the nature of systems, of their components, and of the relations or "forces" between them. The system components need not be material; for example, system analysis may be applied to a commercial enterprise where components such as machines, personnel, buildings, money and *good will* of customers make up the components of the system (von Bertalanffy, 1967). Von Bertalanffy (1967, pp. 69-70) describes some principal features of systems:

> Among systems features are multivariable interaction, maintenance of wholes in the counteraction of component parts, multilevel organization into systems of ever higher order, differentiation, centralization, progressive mechanization, steering and trigger causality, regulation, evolution toward higher organization, teleology and goal-directedness in various forms and ways, etc.

The general system theorists posit that, though every living system and every level is obviously unique, there are important formal identities of large generality across levels. (Some evidence for this assertion is reviewed in a later section dealing with the posited carcinogenic effect of information load-mismatch in non-CNS somatic structures: cells, skin, breast, colon, etc.). However, it is appropriate here to present some of the evidence for this viewpoint.

Cross-level similarities in information processing apparently exist at the CNS and non-CNS levels. It seems reasonable to assume that both CNS and non-CNS structures acquire an enhanced ability to organize the environment with increasing experience. That is, apparently all physiological structures are built up with experience and each structure organizes subsequent experiences in related contexts. Each structure specializes in passing information from its own special environment; e.g., the immunological system passes information from antigens, bacteria and viruses, the skin from solar radiation and atmospheric elements, etc.

Processes analogous to the orienting response and habituation seem to obtain in non-CNS structures. For example, if a given immunological system is highly experienced or developed and it is subsequently exposed to an ordinary antigen or virus, it shows only a minimal orienting response accompanied by a fairly low level of development of defensive orienting responses. It quickly dispatches the appropriate antibodies, macrophages, etc., to destroy the foreign agent, and quickly returns to some baseline resting level of activity. However, if the immunological apparatus perceives a highly novel, exotic bacillus or virus, its orienting response is likely to be enhanced compared to the former condition, and its effecting appropriate defensive responses occupies a longer time period.

Similarly, a cardiovascular system with little development or experience (exercise), upon exposure to a modicum of exercise will show a relatively large *orienting response* consisting of increases in blood pressure, pulse and stroke volume, and heart rate. But if the system has a relatively high development of structure and/or experience which has accrued with regular exercise, it shows a smaller orienting response to the same exercise regimen. In each of the aforementioned instances, activity within a non-CNS structure or system is seemingly inversely related to the degree of development or experience in the structure (system).

There is evidence that the concepts of an "optimal level of information flow and/or stimulation for organized function," and "protective inhibition" not only obtain at the CNS-organism level of analysis but also at CNS cellular and organ levels. Thus, it is possible to overload a cell specialized for the transmission of information—a neuron—by increasing the rate of input of electrical impulses to it until finally its transmission disorganizes or breaks down. A review of relevant research indicates that there is as yet no agreement as to how neurons code information; it is not possible therefore to make a direct translation from neural impulses per second to bits per second. However, if the not too-unreasonable, first-order assumption is made that there is correlation of some sort between the number of impulses and the number of bits per second, input-output performance curves of neurons in units of impulses per second may be assumed to have a similar shape to curves calculated in bits per second. In many neurophysiological studies, the rates of stimulation of cells were altered and the outputs measured electronically. Granit and Phillips (1956) studied the responses of a Purkinje cell of the cerebellum to increasing rates of stimulation. They found that the output rate followed the input rate up to about 180 impulses per second, but when stimulation was increased to about 280 impulses per second, the output of the cell fell to 30 per second.

Input-output performance characteristics of organ systems have also been studied, the units in such researches also being impulses rather than bits per second. Function of the complete visual tract, an entire organ system, was investigated by Jung and Baumgartner (1955), who made microelectrode recordings from the optical cortex in cats stimulated by light impulses of constant duration but various rates of flicker. Concerning what was called "B-Type" reactions in the optical cortex, they made the following observations: the discharge rate increases from about twenty-two per second when four flashes per second were given to the cats, up to a maximum of twenty-five per second when seven flashes per second were given. On further increase of flash frequency the rate of discharge impulses diminished, so that at ten flashes per second, it was eighteen; at eighteen flashes per second, it was fifteen; and at fifty flashes per second, it was six.

The implications are: that both CNS and non-CNS structures process information from the environment; that each structure has some optimal range of information processing for organized function; and that structures at any level of organization within the hierarchy of structures may experience information overload and/or information underload. The former is more likely to obtain in structures with minimal experience or development, and the latter condition more likely in highly developed (phylogenetically evolved) or experienced structures.

THE CONCEPT OF EMERGENCE

Premise 14: Complex systems manifest emergent characteristics which are more than the sum of the characteristics of the simpler units which make up the complex system.[13]

A clear-cut illustration of "emergents" can be found in a comparison of three electronic systems (Miller, 1973). One of the systems—a wire connecting the poles of a battery—can only conduct electricity, which heats the wire. If several tubes, condensers, resistors, and controls are added, the new system can become a radio, capable of receiving sound messages. And if dozens of other components, including a picture tube and several other controls are added, the system may become a television set which can receive pictures as well as sound. The latter two systems are not just more of the same. The third system has emergent capabilities the second system did not have, emergent from its special design of much greater complexity, just as the second system has capabilities the first lacked. But there is nothing mystical about the images on the TV screen. They are the output of a system which can be completely explained by a complicated set of differential equations representing the characteristics of each of the set's components.

In living systems, the problems of emergents gains added complexities and is often discussed as the issue of "reductionism" versus "emergence." Because of the success of the Watson-Crick model of DNA structure in explaining so many fixtures of the living system, the recent elucidation of the genetic code, and the impressive body of knowledge generated about the mechanics of information processing and control in living systems, many life scientists (perhaps the majority) believe that all life can be reduced to the laws of physics and chemistry. Such a view essentially claims that quantum mechanics is the underlying theoretical basis of life because all of chemistry can, in principle, be deduced from quantum theory (Gatlin, 1972). The assumption is that the mathematical theory underlying biology now exists and "all that is left to do is to fill out the handbook" (Gatlin, 1972).

Quantum mechanics is the law that must be demonstrated to be relevant and applicable to living systems. Von Neumann (1955) has shown conclusively that quantum mechanics forms a complete mathematical system which is unique under its postulates. Two physicists, Elsasser (1958) and Wigner (1967) have attempted to find out, by the responsible techniques outlined by Pattee, if the living system does in fact obey this fundamental law. Both, however, have met with serious difficulties, and neither believes that quantum mechanical laws are adequate to explain the living system. Both have postulated the existence of higher "biotonic" laws which govern living systems (Gatlin, 1972).

Precisely what these new biotonic laws are no one seems to have stated clearly yet. Crick (1967) has labeled this position "neo-vitalism." (A neo-vitalist is one who holds vitalistic ideas but does not want to be called a vitalist). But Crick is apparently missing the essential point of the neo-vitalists which is that the existing laws of physics and chemistry may well turn out to be inadequate to describe the living system for the same reasons that the laws of Newtonian mechanics were inadequate in dealing with the interior of the atom.[14] In no way does such a position imply a belief in supernatural or mystical forces.

However, a number of reputable physicists have voiced opposition to the reductionist position, charging that molecular biologists too often claim that cells obey the laws of physics without citing any laws of how they operate. Pattee (1967) summarizes the situation:

> Although the chemical bond was first recognized and discussed at great length in classical terms, most physicists regarded the nature of the chemical bond as a profound mystery until Heitler and London qualitatively derived the exchange interaction and

showed that this quantum mechanical behavior accounted for the observed properties of valency and
stability. On the other hand, it is not uncommon to
find molecular biologists using a classical description of DNA replication and coding to justify the
statement that living cells obey the laws of physics
without ever once putting down a law of physics or
showing quantitatively how these laws are obeyed by
these processes.

A more forceful spokesman for the "anti-reductionist" viewpoint
is Michael Polanyi (1967, 1966). He draws directly on the laws of
information theory in his attempt to explain why quantum mechanics
is inadequate to explain the living system. He believes that because
the living system is a machine, it is irreducible to the laws of physics
and chemistry. He suggests that we cannot understand an information
processing machine, or any machine for that matter, merely from a
description of its hardware. The vast majority of people who use
computers, for instance, study only the operational principles governing the behavior of the machine and, above all, the languages which
can be used in conversing with it.

Polanyi suggests that there are higher operational principles
governing the design and function of a machine which cannot be
deduced from a description of its hardware, no matter how accurate
and detailed the description. In addition he says that the operation of
a machine is governed by "boundary conditions" which are not in any
way determined by the structural laws of chemistry and physics,
adding that these operational principles and boundary conditions
constitute a more fundamental definition of the machine than its
hardware and circuitry. He postulates a hierarchy of control whereby
the higher operational principles take precedence over the lower laws
of physics and chemistry which oversee the operation of the hardware
in much the same manner as does a technician whose responsibility is
restricted to keeping the machinery operating. Moreover, Polanyi
suggests that the higher operational principles fix the boundary
conditions. Polanyi's unique statement of the anti-reductionist position thus makes an attempt to outline what these "new" laws beyond
the presently known laws of physics and chemistry might be (Gatlin,
1972).

Both viewpoints agree that the living system may be regarded as a
machine that stores and processes information. The reductionist can
be likened to a systems expert whose objective is a detailed description of the computer's hardware (i.e., structure). Such knowledge is
clearly indispensable, and it is not surprising that this is the first
aspect of the living system to receive concentrated effort. However,
such a nuts-and-bolts approach may not be sufficient to explain and
describe the living system.

Gatlin (1972) points out that the crux of the problem lies in the
usage of the inexact phrase, "the laws of physics and chemistry." If

one includes information theory, game theory, and related areas of mathematical knowledge within the laws, then the present writer has reductionist leanings. However, it is difficult at present to broaden the scope of the phrase to include additional theories. The laws of physics are constantly evolving, and the laws of today that are "true" will take their place as special restricted cases under the more general laws of tomorrow.

Gatlin further explains that in theoretical physics mathematical knowledge is applied to the understanding of the physical universe. The beginning student learns to apply calculus in Newtonian mechanics. In quantum mechanics, he applies his knowledge of the solution of partial differential equations. Thus that particular portion of the body of mathematical knowledge which is applied to the description and prediction of the physical system becomes a part of the laws of physics. In general, one does not consider unapplied mathematical knowledge a part of these laws. For example, the tensor calculus first developed by Ricci and Levi-Civita was not a part of the laws of physics until Einstein applied it.

Gatlin suggests that since the theoretical foundations of biology are incomplete, there exists a body of mathematical knowledge, developed or undeveloped, which awaits application to the living system. Information theory, game theory and related areas constitute such a body of knowledge; this body is still expanding and will perhaps be unified one day, eventually becoming a part of the laws of physics. It cannot reasonably be considered as such now because it is largely unapplied and even incomplete in its mathematical development. If the scope of the phrase "the laws of physics and chemistry" is used in the more conventional sense, i.e., is limited to mathematical knowledge which has already been applied in detail to the physical universe, then the present writer has anti-reductionist (emergentist) leanings.[15]

SYNOPSIS OF THE PREMISES

The premises outlined in these chapters are intended to lay the foundation for the metaphysical position to be taken in subsequent chapters vis-à-vis the structure and function of nature. Premise 1 points out that increments in experience are represented somatically by structures (including physiological and psychological) which are built up and which, in turn, actively organize subsequent experience(s) in related environmental contexts. Premise 2 presents supporting literature for the idea that structures process information (used in the current mathematical sense of the term) from stimulus events and configurations. That information varies in quantity and in reference is the main point of Premise 3. Premise 4 makes a case for the proposition that the brain has a limit as to the rate of information it can accept. Premise 5 asserts that the amount of information processed by the brain and/or CNS is generally synonymous with the level/amount of physiological activation in the brain and/or CNS.

Premise 6 provides evidence for the view that the brain has an optimal range of information flow for organized function; information flow above or below this optimal range effects a disorganization of perceptual, cognitive, and behavioral functions and the experience of anxiety.

Premises 7 and 8 present support for the proposition that the brain has a variety of hierarchically organized, but imperfectly coupled controls (including brain controls effected during sleep), which operate to effect homeostatic changes in its own information input when information flow falls outside the optimal range needed for organized perceptual, cognitive, and behavioral function. The concept of automatization and its relation to development and/or experience is described in Premise 9. Premise 10 argues that automatization is a central dimension in evolution and necessary condition for the development of perceptual-motor and cognitive skills. Automatization of attention is also argued to be at the core of the experience of boredom, loneliness and ennui. Premise 11 points out that some attempts at rectification of the low intensity of consciousness associated with automatization of attention are often adaptive for self and society and are often associated with the production of great works of art and science, while some are maladaptive for self and society (e.g., violence and hyperactivity, hallucinations and delusions).

Premise 12 continues the emphasis on development, asserting that structures with greater experience/development are more predisposed to disorganization of function upon exposure to information-poor environments, and vice versa. That Premises 1-12 apply not only at the CNS-organism level, but also at CNS and non-CNS sub- and supra-levels of structure within the hierarchy of structures in nature is the focus of Premise 13. Premise 14 outlines the concept of "emergence" as applied to complex systems and suggests that the author's philosophical leanings are reductionistic or anti-reductionist "emergentist" depending upon the definition of the phrase "the laws of physics and chemistry."

Chapter 4 The Mismatch Hypothesis of Carcinogenesis: Experimental Support

There is a sharp disagreement among competent men as to what can be proved and what cannot be proved, as well as an irreconcilable divergence of opinion as to what is sense and what is nonsense.

Eric Temple Bell,
Mathematician

SYNOPSIS OF MISMATCH HYPOTHESIS

Chronic information underload is considered the *sine qua non* of carcinogenesis. Structures may realize a chronic information underload state via two different routes: (1) most adulthood-onset cancer is posited to be associated with a chronic mismatch between relatively high structural needs for information flow for organized function and amounts of information provided by ordinary, habituated-to environments, (2) less frequently in adulthood-onset cancers, and more frequently in childhood-onset cancer, as well as in cancers initiated by exposure to certain environmental carcinogens (radiation, chemicals, etc.), structures experience chronic information *overlaod*. In many childhood-onset cancers, minimally developed somatic structures are easily overwhelmed by even ordinary informational environments. In some adulthood-onset cancers, chronic and/or even short-term exposure to unusually high information loads from certain environmental sources (radiation, chemicals) may induce a condition of severe information overload, even for stuctures with average to above-average levels of development. In both instances, chronically overloaded structures initiate protective information-reducing mechanisms which effect a compensatory information underload state. If the latter condition is chronic and/or severe enough that information flow is below optimal levels for organized function and viability of the structure is compromised, carcinogenesis may be called into play to rectify the chronic information underload.

I posit two main optimal information-load mismatch components in carcinogenesis: a CNS component which effects a generalized nonspecific modulating influence (enhancing carcinogenesis with

50

information underload, inhibiting cancer with information overload); and a non-CNS component which is specific in influence and which determines the initial somatic site of cancer. I suggest that whether carcinogenesis is initiated, and in which structure, as well as it's temporal and spatial dynamic, is the result of interplay between "psychosomatic" influences in CNS and non-CNS structures.

CNS OPTIMAL INFORMATION LOAD-MISMATCH AS A NONSPECIFIC MODULATOR OF CARCINOGENESIS

Statement of the Problem

The belief that psycho-physiological-emotional factors may be involved in the etiology of carcinogenesis has a long history. In the year 2 A.D. the Greek physician Galen made the observation that melancholic women were more prone to cancer than were sanguine women. During the eighteenth and nineteenth centuries frequent mention was made of the significance of emotional and personality factors in the etiology of neoplastic disease. A number of studies dealing with psychosomatic aspects of cancer have been reported in the literature during the past thirty-five years (Miller and Jones, 1948; Bacon et al, 1952; Blumberg et al, 1954; Kissen and Le Shan, 1964; Bahnson and Bahnson, 1964; Aimez, 1972). These studies have been carried out with methods ranging from anecdotal procedures to case histories and psychological testing. The data reported are generally suggestive in implicating emotional and personality variables in the etiology of carcinogenesis, but most of this work with humans can be criticized on methodological grounds (cf. Marcus, 1976). However, while this research has not provided convincing empirical evidence that psychological factors are involved in human carcinogenesis, it has played a role in modifying earlier views of cancer as a strictly autonomous cellular phenomenon and in the current acceptance of a close relationship between carcinogenesis and the functional state of the *entire* organism.

Since controlled empirical work in humans is non-existent, it seems reasonable to review animal work on the effects of psycho-physiological stress on carcinogenesis. There now exists a vast body of literature describing experimental work on animals (Table 1).

At first glance, it would appear that these studies provide contradictory results: some suggest that stress may inhibit malignant tumor growth (24 studies), some yield equivocal results (11 studies), while others report that stress seems to promote tumor growth (40 studies). The complexity of the problem is in part due to the multiplicity of variables which affect host-tumor relationships: age, sex, nutritional status, activity of the host, type of stressor, type of cancer, method of tumor induction, definitions of malignancy and stress (Ader, 1966; Corson, 1965; Peters and Mason, 1979).

TABLE 1. Studies on the Effects of Stress on Carcinogenesis

Facilitation	Inhibition	No Effect
Doderlein 1926 (116)	Rusch & Kline 1944 (154)	Schatten & Kramer 1958 (160)
Deelman 1927 (117)	Muhlbock 1951 (11)	Harvey & Field 1957 (177)
Mackenzie & Rous 1941 (118)	Rashkis 1952 (156)	Ader & Friedman 1964 (178)
Andervont 1941 (8), 1944 (9)	Albert 1956 (133)	Marchant 1966 (179), 1967 (180)
Strong 1945 (121)	Marsh et al. 1959 (158)	Ader 1966 (181)
Petrova et al. 1946 (122)	Lemonde 1959 (159)	Otis & Scholler 1967 (182)
Voskresenskaia 1948 (123)	Schatten & Kramer 1958 (160)	Kaliss & Fuller 1968 (183)
Muhlbock 1951 (11)	Smith & Lazere 1960 (161)	La Barba et al. 1969 (184)
Raushenbakh et al. 1952 (125)	Silverstein et al. 1961 (162)	La Barba et al. 1970 (185)
Nesterova-Kozhevnikova 1951 (126)	Abrams et al. 1961 (163)	Somogyi & Kovacs 1971 (186)
Khaletskaia 1954 (127)	Levine 1962 (164)	
Samundzhan 1954 (128)	Hoffman et al. 1962 (165)	
Olenov 1955 (129)	Newton et al. 1962 (166)	
Finkel & Schribner 1955 (130)	Albert et al. 1962 (143)	
Turkevich 1955 (131)	Gottfried & Molomut 1964 (147)	
Molkov 1955 (132)	Matthes 1964 (196)	
Albert 1956 (133)	Ader & Friedman 1965a (169)	
Reznikoff & Martin 1957 (134)	Newton 1965 (146)	
Lewis & Cole 1958 (135)	Lemonde 1966 (171)	
Kavetski 1958 (136)	La Barba et al. 1970 (172)	
Buinauskas et al. 1958 (137)	La Barba et al. 1971 (459)	
Weder et al. 1959 (138)	Newberry et al. 1972 (173)	
Fisher & Fisher 1959 (139)	Amkraut & Solomon 1972 (151)	
Kavetskii & Turkevich 1959 (140)	Ray & Pradhan 1974 (175)	
Levine & Cohen 1959 (141)	Newberry et al. 1975 (405)	
Echman & Koppe 1961 (142)		
Albert et al. 1962 (143)		
Sing-Mao 1963 (144)		
Newton 1964 (145)		
Newton 1965 (146)		
Gottfried & Molomut 1964 (147)		
Ader & Friedman 1965b (148)		
Ebbesen & Rask-Nielsen 1967 (149)		
Chouroulinkov et al. 1969 (150)		
Amkraut & Solomon 1972 (151)		
DeChambre & Gosse 1973 (152)		
Seifter et al. 1973 (153)		
Henry et al. 1975 (406)		
Riley 1975 (407)		

Primary Variables Influencing Stress Effects on Carcinogenesis

Of the many variables affecting host-tumor-stressor interrelations, a few seem to carry relatively greater weight in influencing the outcome of the interaction.

Manner of Cancer Induction

The tumor may be induced by external agents entering and remaining in the body, or introduced by external intervention such as inoculation or transplantation of tumors, or the tumor may develop spontaneously. While all present antigenic challenges to the host (Kaliss, 1965; Klein, 1966), these challenges are certainly much more subtle for the spontaneous cancer. Work relating stress to the effect on transplanted or induced tumors has been confined to the laboratory rat and house mouse, and these studies primarily have used the nonspecific Walker 256 carcinosarcoma which has a highly variable latent period, death of the host ranging from 14-70 days (Dunham and Stewart, 1953).

Complicating the interpretation of results from studies employing induced tumors are genetic diversities of the hosts—noninbred rats, of several different stocks, that react with an unpredictable variability to an implant antigenically foreign to some degree. Another complication is that the timing of the stressor in relation to the time of tumor implant often makes a difference in enhancing or depressing tumor growth (Jarvey and Field, 1957; Ukolova et al, 1964). In view of the differences characterizing studies of tumors, it seems reasonable to use this dimension as a classification variable in evaluating the effects of stress on cancer.

Tumor Characteristics

Type and/or site of the cancer is a second major variable influencing stress effects on cancer. There are two main classes of tissues which can exhibit carcinogenesis: *epithelial* tissue which refers to the sheet of cells that line body surfaces, from the exposed external facets to the cavities and lumens of the glands; and *mesenchymal* tissue, which refers to nonepithelial cells which migrate and extend between epithelial cells and which effect connective or supporting roles. Cell turnover (degeneration and repair) is much higher in epithelial cells than in mesenchymal cells (von Bertalanffy, 1960). Smithers (1960) has pointed out that 75% of cancers occur in sites where cell turnover is greatest, these being sites in contact with the environment or else subject to relatively greater recurrent stimulation. In view of their differences, it is not surprising that some studies have found that the same stressor conditions show different effects on cancers of epithelial and mesenchymal tissue. Albert (Albert, 1956; Albert et al, 1962) reported that virgin mice of the RIII strain, when kept two in a cage, developed mammary cancer in 80.9% of the cases, whereas those living twenty-four in a cage showed a 22.2% incidence of the tumor. The *opposite* finding was true for malignant mesenchymal neoplasms; leukemia, reticulosarcoma and lymphosarcoma were found to appear more frequently in the mice kept twenty-five in a cage (46.6%) as compared with those living in pairs (7.1%).

Size and Number of Tumors

Size and number of tumors are often-reported characteristics mentioned in the literature. It is important to differentiate these characteristics because often there is little correlation between the effect of a particular stressor on each of these two attributes. For example, Newberry et al (1972) reported a series of experiments dealing with the effects of long-term electric shock stress on rat mammary tumors induced by 7, 12-dimethylbenz[a]anthracene (DMBA). The first study reported a trend for severe stress to inhibit tumor induction as measured by the *number* of palpable tumors. A second study demonstrated that severe shock stress for eighty-five consecutive days produced a significant reduction in the number of tumors. A third experiment applied the same stress for forty days and also found a significantly reduced tumor *count,* while twenty-five-day stress did not significantly influence the *number* of tumors. In no case did the stressor significantly affect average tumor *size.*

Stressor Characteristics

PSYCHOPHYSIOLOGICAL VS. PHYSICAL (INJURY) STRESS. Psychophysiological stress is defined here as optimal information load-mismatch for the CNS, for some temporal interval, in which some optimal range or level of stimulation for organized cortical function is either exceeded or undershot; i.e., when rate of information flow through a given subsystem(s) of the CNS is abnormally high or low relative to some optimal range of stimulation for organized function. Thus, subjecting an animal to electric shock, audiogenic stress, isolation, or protracted forced-swimming are psycho-physiological stressors because each procedure provides an amount of information which is below or above some optimal range of information processing required for organized cortical function.

On the other hand, physical injury stress is associated with relatively longer lasting deleterious effects on information flow and organized function in that structure damage is often involved (e.g., surgical wounding, burns, or lacerations). There is some suggestion, in the literature, that there may be differences between psycho-physiological and physical injury stressors vis-à-vis host-tumor-stressor inter-relations (all other things—chronicity of stress, animal strain, type and/or site of tumor, etc.—being equal). Gottfried and Molomut (1964) reported that whereas surgical trauma *promoted* tumor growth (i.e., a decrease was observed in latent period of tumor growth both in chemical carcinogenesis and tumor grafts, and an increase in the growth rate of the tumors), audiogenic and electric shock stress (presumably carried out on a similar temporal schedule) *retarded* tumor growth (i.e., an increase was observed in latent period of tumor growth and tumor grafts, and a decrease in the growth rate of the tumors).

INFORMATION OVERLOAD VS. INFORMATION UNDERLOAD STRESS. While some forms of psycho-physiological stress (unpredictable environments, accompanied by periodic unpredictable negative reinforcers such as electric shock) effect an *accelerated* rate of information processing, other stress situations (e.g., sensory isolation, quasi-sensory deprivation) involve a *reduction* in the rate of stimulation compared to some normal baseline environment. Information overload and information underload stress apparently have markedly different effects on carcinogenesis, as does the relative intensity and/or chronicity of the stress. Evidence for this claim is extensive and is deferred to a later section.

DURATION OF STRESS. Newberry et al (1972) studied the

effects of long-term electric shock stress on rat mammary tumors induced by DMBA. Severe shock stress applied for eighty-five consecutive days produced a reduction in the number of tumors, higher adrenal weight and lower ovary weights relative to controls. Application of the same stress regimen for forty days also reduced the tumor count, but twenty-five-day stress did not significantly influence the number of tumors.

Age of Host

As discussed earlier, increasing age implies a relatively high development of cognitive (CNS) structure, a relatively low sensitivity to minimal intensity stimulation, and a concomitant susceptibility to experience disruption of organized functioning more from environmental information underload than from information overload, whereas decreasing age implies the converse. While there are no studies in the literature which directly compare the effects of psycho-physiological stresses on cancer in young versus older organisms, there is abundant indirect evidence indicating that younger animals are more susceptible than older ones to carcinogenesis associated with information overload. For example, Richards (1972: 71) reports that it is generally recognized that most tumor-producing viruses (here conceptualized as information) are likely to produce cancer in newborn rather than adult animals. Epidemiological data also indicate that young children living in the moderately polluted greater Los Angeles area show a higher incidence of lung cancer than do older children and adults living in the same environment (Sullivan, 1973). Air pollution is here conceptualized as information overload for the relatively inexperienced lung.

HYPOTHESIS I: ROLE OF THE CNS

The CNS effects a generalized, nonspecific modulating influence on carcinogenesis. In general, chronic information underload (CNS depression, experience of boredom) enhances, whereas information overload (CNS activation, experience of excitement) inhibits carcinogenesis of epithelial tissue in adult animals. These modulating effects are reversed under conditions of extreme (chronicity, intensity) information underload-overload (CNS depression-activation). (Fig. 2).

The latter "paradoxical" effects obtaining with *extreme* levels of CNS information underload/inundation (CNS depression/activation) are associated with the brain's effecting compensatory, homeostatic changes in its own information processing so as to effect a more optimal information processing for organized function. For example, when the brain undergoes extreme information deprivation it effects a compensatory information-inundating, physiologically activating state (hallucinations and/or increased motoric activity) which effects a paradoxical inhibition of carcinogenesis. The information overload and/or CNS activation obtaining with the "switching in" of the compensatory excitatory state has an inhibiting effect on carcinogenesis of epithelial tissue in adult animals. And similarly, under conditions of extreme information overload and/or extremely high CNS activation, the brain switches in a compensatory, protective, *information-reducing*, CNS depressing physiological state which is associated with a paradoxical promotion of most cancers of epithelial tissue.

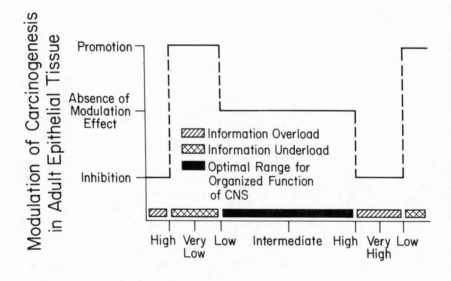

Sensory Information Flow and/or
Physiologic Activation in the CNS

Figure 2

EXPERIMENTAL EVIDENCE FOR THE HYPOTHESIS

The major focus of this section will be a review of direct experimental evidence on the effects of psycho-physiological stress on naturally occurring or spontaneous tumors. Moreover, since spontaneous (as opposed to induced) cancer of epithelial tissue in adult animals is the dominant type of cancer found in nature, the focus of this section will be primarily on the relative effects of information overload and underload psycho-physiological stress on spontaneous cancers of epithelial tissue in adult animals.

With the aforementioned focus, and upon categorization of studies of stress effects on carcinogenesis along the classificatory dimensions described earlier in this presentation, the following results obtain (Table 2).

TABLE 2. Effects of Information Underload/Overload on Spontaneous Cancers of Epithelial Tissue in Adult Animals

Type of Stressor

	Information Overload			Information Underload	
Tumor Inhibition	Andervont	1941,	1944		
	Muhlbock	1951	(exercise)		
	Muhlbock	1951	(crowding)		
	Albert	1956			
	Albert *et al.*	1962			
Tumor Enhancement	Petrova *et al.*	1946		Andervont	1941, 1944
	Turkevich	1955		Strong	1945
	Reznikoff &			Muhlbock	1951
	Martin	1957			
	Henry *et al.*	1975		Finkel &	
				Schribner	1955
				Albert	1956
				Albert *et al.*	1962

Table 2 supports the hypothesis in the following way: tumor inhibition is found with information overload and tumor enhancement with information underload conditions; on the other hand, the four studies finding tumor enhancement with information overload—Petrova et al, 1946; Turkevich, 1955; Reznikoff and Martin, 1957; Henry et al, 1975—employed a condition of *extremely* high information overload.

Information Underload and Overload Stress and Carcinogenesis

Stressors in the respective studies were introduced in such a way that the intensity and chronicity of the stressor condition did not induce an *extreme* level of information overload stress. That is, while the conditions were of moderately long duration, the intensity of the stress was minimized by introducing a certain amount of situational redundancy which served to minimize the moment-to-moment and day-to-day environmental uncertainty. Andervont (1941, 1944) isolated virgin mice into separate cages at 4 weeks and others at 20 weeks of age and the animals were left in the separate cages for the remainder of their natural life. Andervont found that isolated animals developed mammary tumors earlier than did mice housed eight in a cage. Virgins isolated at 4 weeks developed tumors at an average of 9.6 months, while nonsegregated litter mates developed tumors at an average of 11.9 months. Animals isolated at 20 weeks of age had an average age at tumor development of 9.1 months, with the nonisolated animals showing tumors at an average of 10.6 months.

Muhlbock (1951) used Dilute-Brown strain virgin female mice in a test of the effects of crowding and isolation on spontaneous mammary cancer. At 21 days of age, the mice were randomly distributed over 4 types of cage conditions: (1) a zinc cage (37 x 47 x 20 cm.) containing 50 animals; (2) a zinc cage of the same size partitioned into 10 sections, each containing 5 animals; (3) a glass jar (12 x 17 x 15 cm.) containing 5 animals; and (4) a round pot (10 cm. in diameter) containing 1 animal.   Each experimental group contained 90-100 animals, and once distributed over the 4 types of cage conditions, remained in the assigned environment until their natural deaths. Significant differences in the percent incidence of cancer were found among the experimental groups. In the cage housing 50 animals, only 29% developed mammary cancer.   In the partitioned cage, 56% developed tumors, while the groups of 5 animals housed in glass jars showed a 67% incidence.   As in the Andervont study, the isolated animals displayed the highest tumor incidence (84%).   Albert et al (1962) studied 200 7-week-old virgin females; one-half of the animals were kept 2 in a cage, the other half, 25 per cage (cages were of equal size) for most of their life-span and were allowed to die naturally. It was found that the crowded group showed mammary cancer in 8 cases (9.0%), while the uncrowded animals developed the tumor in 56 cases (70.0%). Similar results were reported by Strong (1945) and by Finkel and Shribner (1955).

Muhlbock (1951) investigated the role of moderate physical activity or exercise on the incidence of mammary cancer in DMBA female mice. He placed mice in groups of five in a glass jar (12 x 17 x 15 cm.). An activity wheel was placed in the cage for the experimental group (98 animals); a control group (103 animals) was not given a wheel. It was found that 43% of the mice using the activity wheel (and running several kilometers per night as a group average) succumbed to cancer, whereas the control group without the activity wheel developed cancer in 67% of the cases.

Extreme Information Load-Mismatch Stress and Carcinogenesis

There are several variables which contribute to the relative intensity of a psycho-physiological stressor. One of the more obvious parameters is the *duration* of the stressor; all other variables being equal, the longer a stressor is applied, the more intense it is. Another but more subtle parameter determining stressor intensity is *predictability;* all other variables being equal, the less predictable the stress, the more intense it is (Weiss, 1970; Mehedova, 1974). Weiss (1970) demonstrated, in a series of experiments, that psycho-physiological and endocrinological stress reactions in rats were considerably more severe when the stressor occurred unpredictably than when its occurrence was predicted by a signal. Unpredictable electric shock resulted in more severe stomach ulceration, a greater rise in body temperature, higher plasma corticosterone concentration, more body weight loss, greater depression of food and water intake, and more defecation than did predictable shocks of the same intensity. Such results were obtained when the warning signal was either auditory (tone) or visual (blinking light), and regardless of whether the animal was mildly restrained or free moving. Other variables determining stressor intensity are frequency and amplitude of the stress; in general, all other things being equal, the higher the frequency and amplitude of the stressor, the more intense it is.

Table 2 showed that there are four reports indicating that information overload stress is associated with an enhancement of spontaneous carcinogenesis of epithelial tissue in adult mice. Upon scrutiny of the stressor characteristics employed in the four studies, it is apparent that a good case can be made for the claim for each of these studies having employed a stress condition of *extreme* information overload. Reznikoff and Martin (1957) studied the effects of relatively prolonged, unpredictable electric shock stress on the incidence and age of appearance of mammary tumors in CC_2 mice (a strain normally exhibiting a high incidence of spontaneous mammary tumors). At four months of age, the mice were individually housed in shock cages (5 x 5 x 5 in.). Stressed animals were given daily intermittent shock three times per hour at irregular intervals for periods ranging from six months to more than a year. Treatment was terminated for each mouse when mammary tumors appeared in the animals. It was found that the experimental animals weighed significantly less than the controls, the weight reduction serving as an index of the stress response. While no *significant* differences were found in ages of tumor appearance among shocked and non-shocked animals, tumors appeared considerably earlier in the stressed group (mean = 284 days of age) than for the nonstressed group (mean = 321 days of age).

Soviet scientists have been studying experiential factors in cancer for several decades (Petrova, 1946; Maliugina et al, 1958), but the original reports of these studies are generally unavailable. Description of methodology and results therefore must be gleaned from a few scattered, brief comments found in various secondary sources (La Barba, 1970). The present author could find only two studies in the Soviet literature on the effects of psycho-physiological stress on spontaneous cancers of epithelial tissue in adult animals. Information gleaned from various secondary sources about the characteristics of the stressors employed, indicates that both studies used a stressor paradigm which can be argued to have produced a condition of *extreme* information overload.   Petrova (1946) performed a study which is described by Ivanov-Smolensky (1954), who writes (: 135-136):

> The development of papillomas was observed in some dogs which had been frequently and for considerable periods of time subjected to neuroses; in most of these, in contrast to the experimental animals not subjected to collisions and nervous breakdowns, dissection revealed neoplasms in the internal organs, mainly of a malignant character (cancer of the lungs, of the urinary bladder, and of the thyroid gland . . .) and, in rare cases, neoplasms of a benign character.
>
> The fact that all these neoplasms were found only in the experimental dogs which for years had been subjected to *repeated* and *severe* [author's emphasis] functional nervous traumas, naturally led to the assumption that this coincidence was not accidental, that the first impetus to the development of these diseases was produced by disturbances of the nervous, and above all, of the cortical activity.

Another secondary source (Khayetsky, 1966) reports that Turkevich (1955) found that C3HA mice (in which spontaneous cancer of the mammaries arises in a high percentage of cases) exposed to daily systematic conditioned reflex activity experienced a more rapid development of mammary cancer than controls; the stress condition also resulted in a higher incidence of tumors appearing at earlier ages than in controls. Unfortunately, it is not possible to determine from this secondary source other details of the stressor condition.   However, since there is evidence for the existence of a *general* Soviet stressor paradigm[16] and assuming that the methodology employed by Turkevich (1955) is likely to be quite similar to that described in the available reports, it is plausible to conclude that the Turkevich study probably employed a stressor condition of extreme-level information overload.   This compares with the usual information-overload stress condition used in most other (non-Soviet) investigations, in that the Turkevich stressor condition is long-lasting and introduces extreme environmental unpredictability or uncertainty.

A relatively detailed description of stressor methodology is given in a report by the Soviet investigator Sing-Mao (Sing-Mao, 1963: 1241):

> The floor of the cage was divided into a front and a rear section (platforms) electrically insulated from each other.   Seven seconds before turning on

the electric shock a bell rang on the rear platform
and stopped as soon as the electric shock turned off
(in 23 sec.). After a 1.5 min. interval, a buzzer was
switched on in the front platform of the cage,
following the same sequence as above. Between
five and twelve 4-min. sessions were conducted
daily (for 10 days). The procedure was changed
periodically (bell replaced by buzzer) and the
interval separating two conditioned stimuli reduced
to a few seconds (instead of 1.5 min.). This resulted
in nervous overstrain. The rats were then left alone
for 2-3 days to avoid excessive exhaustion . . . . This
traumatization of the rats' nervous system by neurosis . . . was renewed and continued for 71 days.

Another description of stressor methodology is given in Kavetskii and
Turkevich's (1959) study which points out that periodic, unpredictable
electric shock was used for "overstraining the nervous processes by
often and prolonged action of a conditioned irritator (a bell)." Other
reports by Khaletskaia (1954) and Tereshenko (1958) indicate that
experimental neurosis-conditioning procedures were imposed on mice
in daily sessions for virtually a whole life-time; their stressor was
relatively long term and/or extremely severe.

Henry et al (406) studied the effects of force breeding (immediate
removal of newborn) and social disorder on spontaneous mammary
tumor formation in mice. Force breeding initiated at the sixth month
of colony life led to fighting among the males and to the loss of the
young by cronism (cannibalism and neglect among the females) at the
ninth month. All twelve female colony members developed tumors
during the subsequent five months. On the other hand, tumors
developed in only 8% of the same age study siblings and in 46% of
study breeders maintained under rapid breeding conditions. Since
tumors did not occur in the population cage until its social system
broke down, Henry et al. concluded that the antagonistic social
interaction known to induce various intense neuroendocrine responses
in these colonies may have heightened susceptibility to tumor formation. In explaining their results, Henry et al conjecture:

Some endocrine responses are likely to lead to
tumor formation and others to tumor suppression . . . . What may be happening in . . . studies
(showing tumor suppression) is that, with daily repetition, the rat learns that the aversive experiences
are self-limiting and (the rat) starts to develop
reliable expectations . . . the accompanying emotions change correspondingly, i.e., from depression
to aggression. By contrast our socialized breeding
females may develop a sustained, depressive, pitui-
tary-adrenocortical response because of continued

failure to cope with the social disorder in the colony (associated with the failure to develop reliable expectations, which promotes the emotion of hopelessness).

Thus, the four studies reporting enhancement of spontaneous cancer of epithelial tissue in adult animals may be argued to have employed *extreme* information overload stress conditions. The results support the proffered hypothesis of carcinogenesis. That is, when the CNS is exposed to extreme information overload, it apparently switches in a compensatory, information-reducing mode of information processing to protect itself from excessive stimulation; the latter, compensatory condition of information underload and/or CNS depression promotes carcinogenesis.

Chapter 5 The Mismatch Hypothesis: Correlational Support

Doctor Thomas sat over his dinner
 Though his wife was waiting to ring,
Rolling his bread into pellets,
 Said, "Cancer's a funny thing.

Nobody knows what the cause is,
 Though some pretend they do;
It's like some hidden assassin
 Waiting to strike at you.

Childless women get it,
 And men when they retire;
It's as if there had to be some outlet
 For their foiled creative fire."

W. H. Auden
"Miss Gee"

INDIRECT EVIDENCE FOR THE HYPOTHESIS

In this section, an attempt is made to show the breadth of explanatory utility of the mismatch hypothesis. A broad range of variables is considered in relation to carcinogenesis in adult animals, and the term carcinogenesis is expanded in some instances to include induced tumors of mesenchymal tissue. The review of indirect evidence supporting the hypothesis is not intended to be an exhaustive one; rather, the aim is to provide supplementary evidence in support of the hypothesis.

Phylogeny

Until recently, it was believed that cancerous tumors afflict all living things, including plants, protozoa, invertebrates, and vertebrates, including man. The exciting recent development in phylogeny-cancer interrelations is the suggestion (Dawe, 1968; Dawe, 1969; Sparks, 1969; Sparks, 1972; Good and Finstad, 1969) that it is questionable whether the lumps and bumps or cellular accumulations found in some plants and invertebrates have features that are associated with the malignant tumors of mammals and other vertebrates. According to Sparks (1972), most of the described tumors of invertebrates: (a) appear to be benign; (b) involve hyperplasia or an unusual proliferation of typical cellular components in response to injury or parasites, rather than true neoplasis; (c) possess a cellular makeup consisting of relatively normal recognizable cell types and lacking mitotic figures, features which indicate relatively slow growth; (d) fail to exhibit metastasis, except in some insect tumors; and (e) lack a non-neoplastic, connective-tissue stroma associated with the neoplastic cells.

Moreover, recent cooperative phylogenetic research points out some fundamental relationships between the proclivity for the development of genuine malignant cancer and the relative development of the *nervous* and *immunological* systems. Seemingly, these capacities evolved closely together. For example, genuine malignant cancer appears late in invertebrate evolution with the flatworm, with the propensity for malignancy exhibiting a general increase with increasing invertebrate evolution (e.g., mollusks and insects, especially the fruit fly). However, even in these higher invertebrates, tumors (or presumed tumors) are still rare by vertebrate standards (Sparks, 1972). Coincidentally, the first centralized nervous system appears in invertebrate evolution in the worm, with increasing differentiation of the nervous system evolving in higher invertebrate phyla such as mollusks and insects. And, correlatively, while the roots and rootlets of adaptive immunity probably exist in some higher invertebrates (Good and Finstad, 1969), the full range of adaptive immune reactions appears for the first time in the hagfish and lamprey, the most primitive of the living vertebrates (Finstad, 1969; Barrett, 1974).

Thus, one point of interest in phylogeny-cancer interrelations is the high positive correlation between the relative incidence of malignant tumors and the relative development of nervous and immunological systems. Plants do not make antibodies, do not have a nervous system, and probably do not develop genuine malignant tumors. Single-celled organisms, such as amœba and paramecia, have no nerve cells to conduct information, exhibit no true immunological system capacity, and probably do not develop genuine cancer (Sparks, 1972; Good and Finstad, 1969). The simplest multicellular animals, such as the sponge, have no true nervous or immunological systems, and there are no reports in the literature suggesting cancer tumors in this animal (Sparks, 1972). The first hint of cancer in invertebrates appears in the cœlenterates (jelly fish, or sea anemone) (Korschelt, 1924; Squires, 1965), but the neoplasms are infrequent and their authenticity has often been questioned (Sparks, 1972). Cœlenterates also exhibit the first and simplest type of nervous system found in evolution—the nerve net—which is spatially diffuse and conducts information in a relatively diffuse manner. While no true immunological system has been found in these animals, the possibility of forerunners cannot be totally discounted (Good and Finstad, 1969). The first centralized nervous system appears in the more advanced invertebrates (worms, insects, mollusks, etc.) and it is probably significant that the first genuine cancer tumors found in invertebrates are also exhibited by these animals.

Findings on the phylogeny of cancer provide general support for the hypothesis in the following way. At the core of nervous and immunological system development is the development of memory capacity. The development of an enhanced memory capacity minimizes the amount of information processing from ordinary environments, because much of the information is already in the organism's memory. The result is an attenuation of orienting responses and associated physiological activation. Thus organisms having more phylogenetic experience, or development, and interacting with ordinary environments are conceptualized to be in a state of relative functional information deprivation and/or low physiological activation compared to less phylogenetically experienced organisms interacting with the same environments. That is, the "same" ordinary environment provides less information to the experienced organism because relatively more information is in the CNS and the result is an attenuated rate of information processing and a relatively low physiological activation level.

Ontogeny

As described earlier (Richards, 1972), cancer appears, by and large, in the late or post-reproductive period of life. Thus, findings on the ontogeny of cancer provide support for the hypothesis in a manner analogous to that described for the phylogeny of cancer. That is, the relatively increased experience of the adult organism is associated with a more developed model or memory of the environment. This developed memory minimizes the probability of surprisal or information processing from ordinary, day-to-day environments, because much of the information is already in the adult's memory, and a minimizing of mismatches between expected and environmental stimulation occurs. The result is an attenuation of orienting responses and concomitant physiological hypo-activation in most environmental-organism interactions relative to that obtaining for the child or less experienced organism. These considerations and the finding that cancer is generally a disease of ontogenetically experienced organisms, coincide with the proffered hypothesis which posits that information deprivation and/or CNS depression has a promoting effect on most forms of cancer.

Mental Retardation

Herbert Snow (1893) was the first to record the observation that mentally retarded individuals have a lower cancer rate. Rauf summarized causes of death among mentally ill and mentally deficient populations in England, Wales, Canada and South Africa, contrasting the rates with cancer deaths in the general populations of these countries. Over a four-year period (1965-1970), he noted that cancer caused about 20% of the total deaths in the population, but only about 8% of the deaths among mentally ill and mentally deficient patients. Cleland et al (1971) reported on the causes of death in a segment of the mentally deficient population, the profoundly retarded, over a fifty-four-year period. The causes of death of the retardates, all of whom were residents at the Austin State School, were markedly divergent from the national population; only 4 cancer deaths were observed out of a total of 660 deaths for the period.

While several factors obviously confound interpretation of these reports (the autopsies may not have been routine, age matched controls were not always used, findings are occasionally based on data from single institutions), the conclusion is consistent: mental dysfunction seemingly protects the individual from cancer.

Noting the limitation of previous studies in this area, Achterberg et al (1978) have conducted the most carefully controlled study to date to more clearly define the parameters of the relationship and to provide a detailed breakdown of diagnostic types as they relate to incidence of malignancy. The sample consisted of 3,214 client deaths reported by the Texas Department of Mental Health and Mental Retardation over a 3½-year period (N = 857). Death from cancer in the mentally retarded constituted approximately 4% of all deaths compared to 18% in the general population. Findings were constant across age, sex, race, and geographical location within the state. Institutionalization did not appear to be a contributing factor to the low incidence. Average age of death for retardate cancer victims was 43.7 years, 10 years older than non-cancer clients ($\bar{x}$ = 33). The most intriguing finding involved intelligence score (defined by Stanford-Binet and Wechsler scales), adaptive behavior level (indexed by the Adaptive Behavior Scale [ABS], a classification system based on an individual's communication, self-help, academic, and sensory motor skills), and percentage of cancer deaths. In general, the lower the I.Q. and the ABS level, the lower the percentage of cancer deaths. As the clients approached normal levels of functioning, the cancer incidence also more closely approximated that of the normal population.

Achterberg et al, however, point out that caution is warranted in data interpretation. Profoundly retarded individuals expire much sooner than other retardates ($\bar{x}$ age of death = 19.8, N = 208), particularly when compared with those diagnosed as being mildly retarded ($\bar{x}$ = 44.2, N = 19). Secondly, if the comparison employed is number of all cancer deaths accounted for by a given ABS level, mild and profoundly retarded are approximately equal. Nevertheless, as Achterberg et al point out, the remarkably low incidence in contrast with the general population remains noteworthy; cancer is the leading cause of death from disease in one-to-fifteen year-old children (15% of all deaths). Thus, regardless of the early age of death, especially in the profoundly retarded group, the projected risk of death based on general population figures would be far in excess of the percentages noted in Achterberg et al's study.

Thus, findings on ontogenetic (mental) retardation provide indi-rect support for the hypothesis: at the core of intelligence is memory capacity and the ability to model or predict the environment. Men-tally retarded individuals are presumably not able to form mental models of expected stimulation as well, or as quickly, as their normal counterparts. The result would be an enhancement of irrelevant sensory-information processing at the expense of relevant sensory and cognitive-ideational information upon exposure to ordinary sensory environments. In effect, retarded individuals might be conceptualized to be continually orienting to irrelevant sensory information and consequently they experience *sensory* information *overload.* As a result, retarded brains are not likely in most circumstances to experience sensory information underload; consequently, there is a lower likelihood of initiating a mechanism (i.e., cancer) to rectify sensory information underload. The result is a relatively low incidence of cancer that is not totally explained by a relatively short longevity.

CNS Activating-Depressing Drugs

Effects on assorted cancers

A number of investigations have shown that moderate-to-high dosages of CNS activating drugs inhibit most cancers, and that drugs producing CNS depression facilitate the development of most malignancies. But *extremely* high dosages of both types of drugs often produce the opposite effect on carcinogenesis (in adults). Turkevich and Balitsky (1953) conducted experiments on rabbits with inoculated Broun-Pearce carcinoma and on mice on which Ehrlich's carcinoma was transplanted. The CNS was stimulated by administering phenamine, caffeine and strychnine in small doses; the CNS was depressed by administering sodium amytal. The research results clearly showed that depression of the CNS favored intense development of malignant tumors, while excitation hindered tumor development. Tereschenko (1956) adminis-tered novacaine and showed that the size of metastases increased with the development of an inhibiting process in the cortex of the brain; a dose of adrenalin which produced cortical activation was found to decrease the size of the metastases.

Studies by the Russian investigators Fadeeva (1951) and Kavetskii (1958) beautifully illustrate the importance of level of CNS activation in the modulation of cancer development. Fadeeva examined the variable influence of different doses of amphetamine, a CNS-stimulat-ing drug. While small doses were observed to increase cortical activation, extremely high doses resulted in a paradoxical depression of CNS activation. Related studies by Kavetskii showed the differen-tial effect of varying doses of amphetamines on the development of cancer; his results provide clear evidence for the proffered hypothesis regarding the role of cortical information processing in cancer. Animals given extremely high doses of amphetamines, caffeine or strychnine (which Kavetskii describes as producing supramaximal cortical inhibition and which would be associated with paradoxical CNS depression) showed an enhanced rate and malignancy of tumor development. Animals given small doses of the same drugs, and showing CNS excitation, displayed slower and less metastasizing development.

Effects on breast cancer

Lacassagne (1961) was the first to discover that reserpine, a CNS depressant, promotes the development of spontaneous mammary tumors in mice. Later, Turkevich et al (1965) obtained similar results in rats. Perphenazine, a tranquilizing drug, was administered daily to DMBA-fed rats (1969); it was found that the number and size of the tumors in the treated animals far exceeded those of the control rats. Perphenazine was also given to DMBA-fed rats who underwent ovariectomy and adrenalectomy six days after feeding DMBA. After five months of treatment with perphenazine, seven of fifteen rats developed mammary cancers, whereas none of the eleven control rats receiving saline injections developed palpable tumors. Recent research by Quadri et al (1973) has demonstrated that injection of L-dopa, the immediate precursor of CNS-stimulating catecholamines, for four weeks, into rats bearing carcinogen-induced mammary adenocarcinomas, inhibited growth and caused complete disappearance of some tumors. On the other hand, injection of methyldopa, a CNS-depressing drug which acts by decreasing catecholamine synthesis, resulted in stimulation of mammary tumor growth compared to saline-injected control rats.

More recently, a flurry of epidemiological studies has documented the enhancing effect of reserpine on mammary cancer. Jick et al (1974) reported that routine scanning of data from a survey of hospital inpatients revealed an association between reserpine use and breast cancer; newly diagnosed cases of breast cancer are over threefold in women exposed to reserpine compared with women not exposed. These results stimulated the collection of two other sets of data, both of which supported the original observation. Armstrong et al (1974), in a retrospective study of 708 breast-cancer patients and 1,430 controls with other neoplasms, found an association between breast cancer and the use of CNS-depressing rauwolfia derivatives. The association assumed statistical significance when other neoplasms previously suggested to be associated with reserpine use were removed from the control group. Heinonen et al (1974) also performed a retrospective study of reserpine use in relation to breast cancer; they reported a significant positive correlation between reserpine use and breast cancer.

Effects on liver cancer

Ruddon (1981) describes several studies which suggest that the CNS depressing drug phenobarbital promotes carcinogenesis in liver. In one study, a 3-week exposure of rats to a chemical carcinogen in the diet produced only a small number of hepatomas after several months, but if the animals were subsequently treated with phenobarbital for several months after carcinogen feeding was discontinued, a high incidence of hepatomas was noted. In another study reviewed by Ruddon (1981), rats were fed a non-hepatocarcinogenic dose of a chemical carcinogen for 2 to 6 weeks followed by 70 weeks of dietary administration of phenobarbital. By 72 weeks, many large hepatocellular carcinomas developed in the phenobarbital-treated animals, whereas only a few small tumor nodules were observed in rats not given phenobarbital. (Ruddon points out that phenobarbital produces only a transient and relatively small increase in DNA synthesis in liver; he suggests that perhaps that is all that is needed to *fix* the carcinogenic damage and to allow for the initial proliferation of a damaged clone of cells, i.e. promotion.)

Effects on leukemia

The above discussion should not be taken to mean that reserpine and other CNS-depressing drugs have a consistent cancer promoting effect on *all* cancers. For example, there is some evidence (Goldin et al, 1957; Kruger et al, 1960a; Kruger et al, 1960b)) that administration of reserpine to animals slows the growth of certain experimental tumors, e.g., leukemia. There are several possible explanations for this result: (a) leukemia, being primarily a disease of childhood, could conceivably result from the excessively high sensory information processing and/or physiological activation characteristics of the childhood state. A paradoxical protective CNS-depressing response may then have triggered the leukemia, which then retracted when reserpine was administered (i.e., the extremely high physiological activation was brought down to a more normal level by reserpine). The evidence supporting this view is the Albert et al (1962) finding that leukemia was found to appear significantly more frequently in mice kept twenty-five in a cage as compared with those living in pairs (the opposite was found for mammary cancer); and (b) not all leukemias are associated with or appear during childhood. Some (adult) varieties could conceivably be associated with low CNS physiological activation. In these cases, administering reserpine would produce an extremely low level of CNS physiological activation, which would then produce a paradoxical CNS activation response which in turn might act to increase the abnormally low CNS physiological activation level. This subsequent effect would be a relative normalization of CNS arousal. This line of reasoning would perhaps explain reports such as Karoljow's (1962) of regression of advanced metastasized cancer (adenocarcinoma of the cervix; melanoma of the leg) by inducing insulin coma treatment; i.e., low arousal was made even lower by such treatment, and a paradoxical protective CNS activation response might then have been precipitated which subsequently effected tumor regression.

Endocrine Hormones

The idea that tumors might be influenced by the state of the host's endocrine system was first proposed by G. T. Bateson in 1896, and it is now established that certain cancers are "hormone-sensitive."

Adrenal Hormones

The adrenal glands lie above the kidneys, one on each side. The pituitary regulates the production of adrenal hormones through its adrenocorticotrophic hormone (ACTH). The pituitary normally increases its production of ACTH when somatic organs are induced to function intensely, e.g., during nervous excitement, physical work, or when tissues are damaged (Selye, 1956). ACTH, in turn, stimulates the hormone secretion of the adrenal cortex. According to Selye, the adrenal cortex produces two basic types of corticoid hormones. One type inhibits inflammation; cortisone and cortisol (COL) belong to this group of anti-inflammatory hormones. The other type generally acts in opposite fashion; these pro-inflammatory hormones include aldosterone and deoxycortiscosterone (DOC).

From the standpoint of the proffered hypothesis of cancer induction, the interesting fact about the two types of corticoids is that they often diametrically oppose each other's effects not only on inflammation, but also on CNS activation (and/or sensory information processing) *and* on carcinogenesis. Selye (1956) reported that the epilepsy-like convulsions induced by CNS stimulants (metrozol, pictrotoxin) were attenuated by DOC and related pro-inflammatory hormones. Woodbury and his associates (Selye, 1956: 173) discovered that if such convulsions are produced with electric current, their intensity can be diminished by DOC (pro-inflammatory) and augmented by cortisol (anti-inflammatory). Patients have been successfully anesthetized for surgery with a close relative of DOC (Selye, 1956:173). There are reports indicating that patients taking anti-inflammatory hormones such as COL or ACTH develop a sense of extraordinary well-being and buoyancy, with excitement and insomnia, not unlike that produced by amphetamines and other CNS stimulants. Forsham (Selye, 1956: 174) also pointed out that ACTH and cortisone produce heightened perception in many individuals. Thus, in general, it would appear that DOC and related pro-inflammatory adrenal hormones resemble in many of their actions the tranquilizing agents (chlorpromazine and reserpine), while cortisol and related anti-inflammatory hormones mimic in many ways certain CNS stimulants such as amphetamines. Finally, there is evidence showing that it is possible to inhibit the growth of certain cancers by treatment with large doses of anti-inflammatory hormones (Selye, 1956: 226). ACTH and COL have proved to be particularly effective in slowing down lymphatic cancers and certain leukemias. Thus, indirect evidence is provided for the hypothesis, in that high CNS activation and/or sensory information processing effected by the administration of anti-inflammatory endocrine hormones generally results in a diminution of some cancers.

Other supporting evidence is reported associations between the development of certain cancers and concomitant adrenal insufficiency (cf. Viewig et al, 1973). For example, Trainen (1963) studied the role of adrenal imbalance in skin carcinogenesis. Hydrocortisone (an anti-inflammatory hormone) was tested separately on the initiating and promoting phase and for excessive adrenal action; adrenalectomy (with subsequent reimplantation of isologous adrenal tissue at the end of the required period) was tested for deficient adrenal action. While the initiating phase remained unchanged by either form of added treatment, the promoting phase was strongly inhibited by hydrocortisone feeding and greatly enhanced by adrenalectomy.

Studies of high altitude stress effects on carcinogenesis provide indirect supporting data for the posited effects of adrenal hormone on carcinogenesis (Tromp, 1974). Exposure to high altitudes is often observed to inhibit certain cancers. Warburg (1926) exposed rats having implanted Jensen sarcoma to a gas mixture containing 5% oxygen (simulating an altitude of 12,000 meters) for forty hours and found that the tumors became markedly necrotic. Campbell and Kramer (1928) repeated the experiment at a simulated altitude of 5,100 meters and found that the growth of inoculated Jensen's rat sarcomas was markedly inhibited. Sundstroem and Michaels (1942) observed regressions in Walker tumors in all experimental series kept at 360 mm. Hg atmospheric pressure (about 6,000 meters altitude); the authors attribute their results to stimulation of adrenal function by the reduced oxygen pressure of high altitudes which change the level of circulating corticosteroids in the blood. The importance of the adrenal gland was suggested by the finding that adrenalectomy of tumor-bearing rats stops further regression after low atmospheric pressure treatment (in fact, the tumors were reported to start growing again).

Thyroid hormone

Thyroid hormone has also been implicated as a retardant of certain cancers. Loeser (1954) has reported the following findings: (a) more obese persons (hypothyroid function) acquire cancer, and their death rate is higher; (b) hyperthyroid patients seldom suffer from cancer; (c) after partial thyroidectomy, a greater number of women develop breast or genital cancer; and (d) administration of thyroid hormone is often observed to slow down cancer growth in the genitals and breasts. These results provide support for the hypothesis, because increased thyroid function is associated with enhanced CNS activation and/or information processing. These studies provide evidence suggesting that CNS activation or information overload retards most types of cancer of epithelial tissue.

Autonomic Nervous System Activation

The work in recent decades has shown that the autonomic nervous system is more than an efferent channel supplying the viscera; Hess recognized as early as 1925 that alterations in autonomic activity are associated with changes in cerebral cortical functions. Procedures leading to increased *sympathetic* discharges are accompanied by cerebral excitation, increased activity and tone of the striated muscles, and behavior arousal. Conversely, increased *parasympathetic* activity is associated with decreased cortical activation, a lessening of somatic action, and a diminution of muscle tone. These general effects of sympathetic and parasympathetic stimulation led Hess to distinguish the ergotropic (work-associated) and trophotropic (rest-related) systems, respectively.

There is a small body of evidence in support of the hypothesis which posits that activation of the sympathetic (ergotropic) system is associated with tumor regression, whereas activation of the parasympathetic (trophotropic) system is associated with tumor enhancement. A report by Puzhak (1964) points out that in many patients with malignant tumors the normal activity of the sympathetic-adrenal system is impaired, and the quantity of adrenalin in the blood is reduced. Puzhak also reports that his own research has determined that the process of cell division in the healthy organism is regulated, in the main, by the parasympathetic nervous system; the sympathetic (as well as the sympathetic-adrenal system) system inhibits the process. Proceeding from the assumption that a malignant growth is in one way or another connected with damage of the activity of the sympathetico-adrenal system, Puzhak injected a 0.1% solution of mesaton, a sympathomimetic substance, into white rats with an inoculated sarcoma M-1 once a day for ten days. The injection caused a marked decrease of mitotic activity in the tumor tissue, amounting in some instances to 50%; the same was achieved with regard to the mitotic activity of the epithelial cells of the cornea of the eye in the same animals. Puzhak thus concluded that the effect of the sympathomimetic substance upon the adrenergic biochemical systems of sarcoma tumor cells is the same as the effect in the corresponding cells of normal tissues. In other studies of autonomic function, Kissen (1969) found that lung cancer patients, according to a self-report inventory, rate themselves as having lower levels of autonomic activity. Kissen and Rao (1969) found that cancer patients, compared to control patients, show less initial levels of adrenergic response at the time of admission to the hospital.

Indirect studies of autonomic function via stimulation and lesion of brain structures such as the hypothalamus and cerebral cortex also support the hypothesis. Electrical stimulation of the posterior hypothalamus causes a sympathetic discharge with a demonstrable release of adrenalin and nor-adrenalin by the adrenal medulla, while lesions of the posterior hypothalamus decrease sympathetic activity (Gellhorn et al, 1956; Gellhorn and Kiely, 1973). On the other hand, stimulation of the anterior hypothalamus elicits parasympathetic discharges, while lesions of these areas decrease parasympathetic activity. In general, the two systems are characterized by mutually reciprocal relations, i.e., with increasing excitation of the ergotropic system there is an increasing inhibition of the trophotropic system and vice versa. Khayetsky (1963) reported that lesions of the anterior hypothalamus, which would result in ergotropic or sympathetic nervous system dominance, inhibited tumor growth on subsequent introduction of the carcinogen DMBA. Ukolova et al (1964) reported that chronic, predominantly-posterior, hypothalamic stimulation in albino rats prior to transplantation inhibited growth of a transplantable sarcoma.

Similar supporting evidence exists from lesion studies of the cerebral cortex. There is much evidence that stimulation of posterior cerebral cortex results in enhanced physiological activation and/or increased sensory information processing (Pribram and Melges, 1969; Spinelli and Pribram, 1966), and that lesions of posterior cerebral cortex result in depressed physiological activation and/or depressed sensory information processing (Luria, 1959; Luria et al, 1966). On the other hand stimulation of frontal cerebral cortex results in lowered physiological activation and/or sensory information processing (Spinelli and Pribram, 1966; Pribram, 1967) and lesions of frontal cortex (Luria et al, 1966; Pribram, 1969) generally result in enhanced physiological activation and/or enhanced sensory sensitivities. As in hypothalamic function, the two systems are characterized by mutually reciprocal relations, i.e., with increasing excitation of the posterior cortex (ergotrophic dominance) there is increasing inhibition of the frontal (trophotropic) system, and vice versa.

Now with respect to cerebral cortex function and cancer, West (1954: 92-93) has observed in many patients that frontal lobotomy, which would result in posterior-cortex dominance and an enhanced level of CNS physiological activation, not only slows tumor growth, it may at times produce definite tumor regression. In addition, he mentions that several other neurosurgeons who had observed the same pheonomenon have described some of these cases at various scientific meetings. According to the proffered hypothesis, lesions of the posterior cerebral cortex should often be observed to *enhance* most types of carcinogenesis found in adult organisms, but no studies or observations along these lines have been reported.

Psychosis-Cancer Interrelations

The coincidence between lung cancer and psychosis is not rare, and has been mentioned in the literature frequently (Hoffer, 1970; Brain et al, 1951; Charatan and Brierly, 1956). Cancer specialists know they should examine the lungs when a middle-aged man becomes psychotic. Brain et al's (1951) four cases of lung cancer all had mental changes (leading to dementia in three). A study by Charatan and Brierly (1965) reported three cases of bronchial cancer who were also psychotic; in two patients, the psychotic symptoms preceded the cancer symptoms, and in one of these the symptoms occurred fourteen months after the initial appearance of cancer. Brain and Wilkinson (1965) reported that eleven to nineteen cancer patients exhibited mental changes, chiefly dementia.

Of more relevance to the proffered hypothesis of carcinogenesis is a body of research literature on cancer and schizophrenia. Josephy (1949) analyzed causes of death in a Chicago State Hospital; he found that cancer occurred less frequently in mental patients than in the general population. In tabulating cancer incidence as a function of mental disease categories, White (1929) found that there was approximately a 13% incidence in paranoids, but only a 4% incidence in nonparanoid patients. Lewis (1936) examined the relationship of cancer to various forms of schizophrenia. The subgroups catatonia and hebephrenia (commonly called nonparanoid schizophrenia) frequently had atrophy of tissue, hypoplasia, and fibrosis, but rarely had cancer. On the other hand, paranoid schizophrenics frequently had hypertrophy, hyperplasia, and cancer.[17] These findings were corroborated by Schefflin (1951) in a different group of institutionalized psychotics. In examining all the records of patients dying between 1928 and 1942 at Worcester State Hospital, he found that the incidence of cancer in schizophrenics is about half that of the general population (matched for age range) and occurs at a later age. Upon differentiating schizophrenics into subtypes, it was found that nonparanoids showed a decreased incidence and death rate from cancer, while paranoid schizophrenics had about four times the incidence compared to the general population at ages forty-five to fifty-four. Cancer in this latter group appeared earlier in life and showed extremely uncontrolled growth patterns. West (1954: 93) has documented an extremely malignant cancer growth pattern in paranoid schizophrenia:

> One of the very "fastest" cases we have ever had was in a young paranoid schizophrenic who had lymphosarcoma. These tumors can almost always be depended upon to respond, at least for a short time, to X-ray therapy, cortisone, or nitrogen mustard, but in this patient the neoplasms extended with unbelievable rapidity, in spite of intensive treatment. Among our longest survivors, we have several representatives of the advanced disintegrated (presumably nonparanoid) schizophrenic. After a while one becomes quite impressed with the apparent reciprocal relationship between psychosis and cancer. As the psychosis becomes more apparent (presumably hallucinations, delusions, and disorganized thinking increase), the cancer regresses or remains quiescent, and as the psychosis is treated and the patient thus returned to his conflict with reality, the malignancy resumes its activity. It seems as if the individual is determined to "get away from it all" one way or the other.

In a recent study of cancer-psychosis interrelations, Achterberg et al (1978) studied 2,387 client deaths reported by the Texas Department of Mental Health and Mental Retardation. Death from cancer in the mentally disturbed population constituted approximately 4% of all deaths as contrasted with 18% of deaths from cancer in the general population. Findings were constant across age, sex, race and geographical location within the state; institutionalization did not appear to be a contributing factor in the low incidence. The investigators noted that within diagnostic categories, differences in cancer mortality percentage were significant: they were exceptionally low (absent) in catatonics and relatively higher in paranoid schizophrenics, thus replicating previously described studies. Findings on enhanced incidence and mortality from cancer in paranoid schizophrenia, and the reported reciprocity relationships between cancer and exacerbations of psychotic behavior (hallucinations, delusions), conform to the proposed hypothesis of CNS activation-cancer interrelations: in the pre-morbid state, the low physiological activation, preparanoid schizophrenic may be conceptualized to experience a chronic, functional sensory deprivation in most of his interactions with ordinary sensory environments. His brain attempts to compensate for this state of information underload and/or low CNS activation by producing psychotic behaviors such as hallucinations and delusions, since these behaviors are associated with an enhancement of physiological activation and/or sensory information processing. At times, the production of cancer (the production of endogenous information) precedes the onset of psychosis; at other times it follows. When the psychotic behavior is most intense or prominent (temporary episodes of hallucinations, delusions) general physiological activation and/or sensory information processing is enhanced and extant tumors recede or diminish. With treatment (most often, tranquilizing drugs), the intense physiological activation subsides to normal or below-normal levels, waking behavior and perception is relatively normalized or subnormalized, and the malignancies return to compensate informationally for the once-again relatively low levels of physiological activation. The nonparanoid schizophrenic, on the other hand, is relatively immune to cancer, and its associated informational "value," because he is already processing an abnormally high level of information and/or he is experiencing an abnormally high level of CNS activation. The relatively enhanced information processing at the level of the CNS results in a compensatory, information-reducing response, so that hypoplasia and tissue atrophy, rather than hyperplasia and cancer, frequently obtain.

The Cancer Personality

The literature on the cancer personality is vast. It is filled with many original and arresting conceptualizations of the role of psychological factors (Gengerelli and Kirkner, 1954) and personality predispositions in the development of cancer. It is also characterized by a plethora of methodological difficulties (cf. Marcus, 1976; Perrin and Pierce, 1959); most studies usually have been attempted retrospectively (Blumberg et al, 1954; Booth, 1964; Cobb, 1952; Cutler, 1954; Bahnson and Bahnson, 1965; Greene et al, 1956; Blumberg et al, 1956; Bahnson and Bahnson, 1969; Davies et al, 1973) and with the inadequate, and probably inappropriate, tools of inquiry that are presently used in most psychological research. Attempts at sophisticated methodology have not always succeeded in achieving a high degree of objectivity, and at times appear to have outstripped the realities of the experimental situation (Crisp, 1970); for example, studies have required that patients not know that they have cancer, and it seems likely that some investigators have on occasion been over-concerned with this. Such barriers to communication might profoundly influence the nature of the communication between interviewer and subject. Another controversial point is the conceptualization of "personality." Mischel (1968, 1973) has pointed out that diverse data challenge and undermine the central assumptions of the traditional trait approach to personality (i.e., that traits, states, motives, etc., exert generalized and enduring effects on behavior, more or less independently of stimulus conditions). A third methodological difficulty is one of ascribing any obtained personality differences between cancer patients and control groups to cause or effect. The mechanism of denial, for instance, probably is vital for the person with a developing awareness that he or she may have cancer (Hinton, 1963; Hinton, 1967).

Pre-morbid personality characteristics of cancer patients

Review of the better-controlled studies suggests that personality predispositions to cancer do exist, and that psychological experiences (e.g., depression, loss of a spouse or job) play a possible role in the onset and course of carcinogenesis (cf. Abse et al, 1974). In general, these studies provide some support for the notion that CNS depression and/or information underload promotes the development of cancer, and vice versa.

Abnormal emotional expression

Kissen (1962, 1963, 1964, 1965a, 1965b) studied large numbers of men admitted to chest hospital units for diagnosis of chest disorders including suspected lung cancer. For the most part, patients were seen in privacy during the week following admission to the units and were not seen post-operatively. In most instances, at the time Kissen studied the patients, the diagnosis had not yet been confirmed, especially where cancer was a possibility. Whatever the suspected diagnosis, most patients were told at this time that they had pneumonia or bronchitis. In no case was the correct diagnosis known to Kissen at the time of the interview. Patients subsequently diagnosed as suffering from any disorders other than cancer served as controls.

Over the years, Kissen repeatedly confirmed his initial finding: that men with lung cancer show impairment of discharge of affect, inadequate outlets for instinctive drives, and low scores on measures of neuroticism (Kissen assumes that the mean neuroticism score measures ability to discharge emotion). Kissen concluded that blocked flow of feeling is a defining, pre-morbid characteristic of the cancer patient.

Kissen's findings get some support from the Greer and Morris (1975) study of patients admitted for breast biopsies. Patients were interviewed before receiving their diagnoses, and were asked about the way they generally expressed anger and other emotions. Patients who never expressed anger or other emotions—or did so not more than twice during their adult lives—were labeled extreme suppressors. Patients who indulged in frequent outbursts of temper or who had never or rarely concealed their emotions were considered extreme expressors. More patients whose biopsies showed cancer were found to suppress all emotions than to express them in normal fashion. However, patients who always gave vent to their emotions also showed a significantly higher incidence of cancer than normal expressors of emotion.

Hagnell's (1965) study provides further support for the notion of emotional expressiveness-cancer interrelations. The report was based on the results of an epidemiological survey of the 2,550 inhabitants of two adjacent rural parishes in southern Sweden; the survey, started in 1947, included an interview during which personality assessment was made on each subject. Ten years later the procedure was repeated and each subject's subsequent medical history was examined. During the follow-up it was found that a significantly high proportion of women who had developed cancer had been originally rated as "substable." Substability (based on the Swedish system of personality assessment described by the Swedish investigator Sjobring) has traits in common with Eysenck's extroversion (Eysenck, 1959; Eysenck, 1962; Kissen and Eysenck, 1962); the substable personality is described as warm, hearty, industrious, sociable, and interested in people. LeShan (1966), in a twelve-year study of the pre-diagnosis emotional life histories of 450 adult cancer patients, noted an extremely high energy level in many of his patients during a period of time in which a situation arose which offered an opportunity for relating to others, and prior to situations fostering generalized depression.

Thus the literature suggests that two pre-morbid personality styles may be associated with carcinogenesis. One type of individual is highly introverted, shows impairment of discharge of affect, inadequate outlets for instinctive drives—the abnormal emotional expressiveness is associated with blocked flow of feeling. The other is highly extroverted, emotionally hyper-expressive, and is extremely energetic (particularly when situations arise offering opportunities for relating to others).

There is evidence suggesting that both types of individuals may be charcterized as having low pre-morbid physiological activation levels and/or high sensory thresholds. In the emotionally hypo-expressive individual, the usual positive correlation between behavioral and physiological activation obtains. Low emotional-behavioral expressiveness is associated with low physiological activation levels (Kissen, 1969; Kissen and Rao, 1969). The CNS of the hypo-expressive individual apparently does not attempt to rectify the low level of information processing and/or physiological activation by engaging the environment in more vigorous fashion than what is considered normal. Rather, the compensatory information flow is accomplished by relatively covert mechanisms, e.g., increased cerebration as in obsessive compulsive ruminations, more sensory information during REM sleep than normal (increased density of REMS), cancer.

On the other hand, for the emotionally hyper-expressive individual, the usual positive correlation between behavioral and physiological activation apparently does not obtain. This is possibly because: (1) waking sensory information flow is *extremely* low so that the relatively covert mechanisms used by the hypo-expressive understimulated individual are simply inadequate to rectify the information deficit; or (2) the waking sensory flow is as low as for the emotionally hyporesponsive individual, but constitutional and/or cultural factors preclude engaging in excessive cerebration or increased activation during REM sleep. Many studies clearly indicate that an extremely high degree of emotional-behavioral responsivity (e.g., highly extroverted adults, hyperactive children) is associated with extremely low resting levels of physiological activation (Eysenck, 1967; Gray, 1967) and high sensory thresholds (Haslam, 1967). The greater emotional expression and/or behavioral intensity is interpreted by many investigators as an attempt by the extremely understimulated CNS to compensate for abnormally low levels of physiological activation and/or information processing in the CNS. For example, hyperactive children and highly extroverted adults generally show significantly lower resting levels of physiological activation (Eysenck, 1962; Cohen and Douglas, 1972; Knopp et al, 1972; Satterfield et al, 1974; Spring et al, 1974) than normally expressive groups matched for age and socioeconomic status. Thus the findings that many emotionally hyperexpressive individuals are predisposed to develop cancer (Hagnell, 1966; LeShan, 1966; Greer and Thomas, 1975), coupled with experimental findings pointing out a negative correlation between behavioral activation (which includes emotional expressiveness) and physiological activation, at the extreme *low* end of the physiological activation continuum, is consistent with the proffered hypothesis that chronic information underload (and/or CNS depression) promotes the development of many types of carcinogenesis.

Depression

There are two major methodological problems characterizing studies relating depression and cancer. The first is that depression is a construct which can be divided along six or seven equally appealing

ategories (Beck, 1967; Lader and Wing, 1969), and the proliferation of
ategories and classification methods reflects the inability of any
,iven diagnostic labeling procedure to neatly compartmentalize de-
ressed individuals (Stern et al, 1970; Stern and Janes, 1973). The
econd methodological problem plagues any study of the association
etween personality and cancer: are the obtained differences between
ancer patients and controls cause or effect? For example, depression
nay be a common accompaniment of a developing awareness by the
ndividual that he may have cancer (Shands et al, 1951). However,
hese methodological problems can be circumvented, to some extent,
y reviewing studies covering as broad a range of categories as
ossible, and studies in which subjects at the time of personality
ssessment were relatively unaware of their illness.

The idea that depression is a common antecedent of cancer has a
ong history. In 2 A.D., Galen considered that melancholic women
uffer from cancer more frequently than sanguine women. In the
iineteenth century, other writers stated similar opinions based on
heir personal observations (Nunn, 1822; Walshe, 1846; Paget, 1870).
More recently, a number of studies have supported the general notion
hat psychological depression may be an antecedent of cancer.
ichmale and Iker (1964; 1965) examined forty women with Papani-
olaou class II changes in their cervical cellular cytology, suspicious,
ut not diagnostic, of cervical cancer, and who were physically fit and
vithout apparent symptoms or signs of cancer. All of the subjects
vere examined psychiatrically one day after cone biopsy and before
he diagnosis was known. A complex multiple assessment of each
voman's state of hopelessness over the previous six months was
conducted, and on this basis, prediction was made concerning the
liagnostic outcome of the cone biopsy. Prediction was accurate for
eight of the fourteen who had cancer and twenty-three of twenty-six
vho did not. The cancer patients scored significantly higher than the
ion-cancer group on the D (depression) scale of the MMPI.

LeShan (1961, 1962) has refined the study of antecedent depression in cancer patients and has introduced the concept of despair with
ts surplus existentialistic and ontological meaning. According to
LeShan, the despairing cancer patient is even worse off then the
severely depressed person because the patient is in despair of himself
and is confronted with a seemingly impossible choice between non-
existence and existence eternally doomed by isolation and rejection.
Munro (1966) has found that a significant excess of mothers of
depressed patients had died of cancer; he postulated the presence of
some underlying familial constitutional factors predisposing to both
cancer and depressive illness. Kerr et al (1969) found a sevenfold
death rate from cancer in males within a five-year period of their
naving presented with depressive illness without evidence of physical
disease at that time. Atypical depression is one of the multiple
conditions determining the development of lymphoma or leukemia
(Greene, 1954; Greene and Miller, 1958).

Although these studies are generally suggestive for implicating

psychological depression in the etiology and pathogenesis of malignan
tumors, virtually all of this work can be seriously criticized in term
of inadequate experimental design, ill-defined independent variables
unvalidated measurement devices, etc. However, it is instructive t
note that the other side of the coin, elation or euphoria, has neve
been reported to be associated with cancer.

There exist some physiological and biochemical data on depressio
which neatly tie in with the proffered hypothesis of modulator
factors in carcinogenesis. The work of Schildkraut and Kety (1967
shows that drugs which cause depletion and inactivation of norepine
phrine in the CNS often produce depression; drugs which increase brai
norepinephrine are associated with behavioral excitement and general
ly have an antidepressant effect in men. Norepinephrine generally ha
the effect of enhancing physiological activation, as measured b
various peripheral and central indices of activation in men an
animals. In addition, there is experimental work showing that unde
hypnosis, if anger on one occasion and relaxation and depression o
another are suggested, the subject shows an ergotropic (sympatheti
autonomic nervous system dominance mediated by norepinephrine
reaction to anger and a trophotropic (dominance of parasympatheti
autonomic nervous system mediated by acetycholine) response t
depression and relaxation as shown by respiratory and metaboli
indicators (Dudley et al, 1964). Electroconvulsive therapy (ECT) whic
has strong ergotropic (excitatory) effects often is used successfully i
the treatment of some forms of depression, implying that certai
depressives may be in a state of abnormally low physiological arousa
which is rectified by the ergotropic excitatory effects of EC
(Gellhorn and Kiely, 1973).

During the 1950s, a number of reports indicated that depressio
often developed in hypertensive patients being treated with reserpin
(Freis, 1954; Achor et al, 1955; Lemieux et al, 1956; Jensen, 1959
Bernstein and Kaufman, 1960). Although many of the reports ar
retrospective and poorly documented, and the relative incidence o
this syndrome cannot be determined from these reports, it is apparen
that CNS physiological depression and the phenomenological experi
ence of depression are associated to some extent. Hall demonstrate
that endogenous depressives appeared to be very insensitive to pai
(Hemphill et al, 1952).   Other studies (Funkenstein et al, 1948
Funkenstein et al, 1949; Alexander, 1961; Jones, 1956) have reported
tendency among psychotic depressives towards prolonged hypotensio
in response to the Mecholyl test, indicating parasympathetic domi
nance and low physiological activation. Kollar (1961), in a review o
literature on the psychophysiology of psychological stress, conclude
that whereas anxiety and aggression seem to be expressed mainl
through adrenosympathetic (ergotropic) mechanisms, depression an
despair (hopelessness) are expressed physiologically, at least in part
through parasympathetic and/or inhibitory-conservatory (trophotropic
mechanisms.

Environmental Event-Life History Data

According to the proffered hypothesis, chronic information underload and/or CNS depression promotes carcinogenesis. Many studies indicate that loss and separation from key objects and significant persons, construed here to effect information underload and/or CNS depression, are important antecedents in the manifest development of cancer (LeShan, 1961; LeShan, 1962; Greene, 1954; Maliugina et al, 1958; Green and Miller, 1958; LeShan, 1959; LeShan and Worthington, 1956; LeShan and Reznikoff, 1960; Meerloo, 1944; Meerloo, 1954; Kowal, 1955; Tarlau and Smalheiser, 1951; Schmale, 1958). On the basis of his own studies (interviews with over 500 patients) and review of the literature, LeShan (1959) writes:

> The most consistently reported psychological factor has been the loss of a major emotional relationship prior to the first-noted symptoms of the neoplasm. It seems to be established that this has occurred more often in cancer patients than in various groups who were used as controls.

In a comprehensive statistical attempt to test the hypothesis of object loss, LeShan and Worthington (1956) reasoned that if their hypothesis were valid, cancer rates should vary in different social groups which had suffered differential losses of important interpersonal relationships. They assumed that the probability of the loss of a crucial emotional relationship in different marital classes would be highest in the widowed group, lower in the divorced group, still lower in the married group, and least in the single group. It was predicted, and subsequently confirmed, that the age-adjusted cancer mortality would be highest in the widowed, next in the divorced, followed by the married and then the singles.

The relationship of bereavement to subsequent high immediate mortality is well-documented. In one epidemiological study (Parkes et al, 1969), cancer was found to be one of the leading causes of death among persons in the first six months of bereavement. Paloucek and Graham (1960) reported that twenty-seven out of forty-nine women had suffered the loss of a strong emotional attachment prior to their development of carcinoma of the cervix. Green (1954, 1958, 1965) observed that leukemias and lymphomas occur in a setting in which the patient deals with loss or separation, with concomitant feelings of sadness, helplessness or hopelessness. Meerloo (1944, 1954), Kowal (1955), Meerloo and Zeckel (1952), and Tarlau and Smalheiser (1951) all emphasized that loss and depression and the inability to handle and express affect following such a situation were characteristic of the cancer patient. Reznikoff (1955) reported a study of fifty women in a clinic for diagnosis of early breast lumps. Psychological assessments were made in the prediagnostic state. Those subsequently found to have breast cancer had reported more sibling death in childhood, and fewer successful marriages.[18]

Thus, studies of life experiences predisposing individuals to cancer suggest that loss of or separation from significant person-object-behavior relationships is associated with the development of cancer. Many of these studies, like those on depression-cancer interrelations, can be criticized on methodological grounds. Thus, since Greene failed to compare his findings with a control group of people without cancer, it is impossible to determine whether loss among his cancer victims was greater than loss in the general population. LeShan's evidence is retrospective. Moreover, there exist some studies (Greer and Morris, 1975; Muslin et al, 1966) which report finding no differences in losses suffered by cancer and non-cancer patients. There is the possibility, however, that the narrow definition of loss employed in these studies may have contributed to the failure to find differences between cancer patients and controls. Thus Muslin et al limited their definition of loss to permanent separation from a person close to the patient. It is possible that different results would have obtained had they employed a broader definition (e.g., Greene's definition was broad, ranging from actual loss of a spouse, sibling or close friend, to loss of a job or home, and finally to the threat of losing any of them).

Pre-Morbid Health in Cancer Patients

Witzel (1970, cf. Fox, 1978) took personal histories from 150 cancer patients and 150 patients with other diseases. He found that cancer patients apparently had experienced superior physical fitness and *better* health in respect to the five years before cancer began (e.g., outpatient status of any kind, 15.3% vs. 44.7%; hospital bed patients, 4.7% vs. 12.7%; number of times fever exceeded 38.5°C, 1.3% vs. 13.3%; illness experienced 28% vs. 57.3%; operations 8.7% vs. 18%). Recently-published autobiographical accounts (Rollin, 1974; Alsop, 1973; Cousins, 1979) of superior general health prior to the manifestation of cancer provide additional support for the Witzel findings. That is, in each case, the authors describe their general level of health to be much better than what is considered normal.

Although other interpretations are obviously plausible, it is possible that these reports provide support for the mismatch hypothesis. Illness may be regarded as a sub-class of information for somatic structures. Superior health and lack of illness suggests the existence of a strong constitution with high development of immunological competence and a kind of functional information underload for the cortex and immunological structures, since extremely good health is associated with internal organismic stability, homeostasis and a lack of change (information). The implication is that too little life-event stress is likely to be associated with carcinogenesis, since illness is a sub-class of life-event change or information.

In general, then, there is considerable evidence which suggests support for the proffered hypothesis of cancer development in the following way: the loss of an important interpersonal, object or behavior relationship is, in the final analysis, the loss or separation from information.   Just as bereavement induces a condition of information underload and/or low physiological activation in the bereaved, so is separation (marital or otherwise) associated with similar effects.   These effects are temporary to the extent that persons, objects, or behavior can be found to substitute for this loss of significant information.   Long-term inability to substitute a new person-object-behavioral activity or relationship (e.g., denial of grief affect, inability to find a new friend, frustration of needs for change in milieu) to replace the experienced loss and resulting information underload seemingly promotes the process of carcinogenesis.   This conclusion is in agreement with the conceptualizations of Bahnson and Bahnson (1965), that "unconsciously the creation of a tumor may be as important and meaningful to the cancer patient . . . as the creation of a plastic form to the sculptor."

CONCLUSIONS

The greater a structure's information processing capacity, the greater the risk for carcinogenesis in one of its parts and/or in structures over which it has some degree of control.   This is because the function of information processing structures is, in the main, the selective *destruction* of the large amount of information in the environment that is irrelevent to the structure's function and viability.   Increments in development (evolution) of such structures are thus necessarily associated with a functional *isolation* of the structure(s) from its environment, including its internal infra-structure environment.   However, structures with low levels of development are also posited to show a relatively high propensity for carcinogenesis, since the correlative information overload, if sufficiently chronic and severe, may initiate information-reducing mechanisms to effect a protective isolation condition; if the latter is chronic enough and effects too low a level of information flow for organized function of the structure, carcinogenesis may be called into play to help rectify the information underload.

Thus carcinogenesis was posited to be linked closely to (1) development and/or evolution of structures having relatively specialized and sophisticated information processing capabilities (2) environmental circumstances associated with a relative isolation of structures from sources of stimulation or information, and (3) structure-environment transactions productive of the experience of isolation, boredom, depression, and loneliness.   Literature review of interrelations of carcinogenesis with phylogeny, ontogeny, mental retardation, CNS activating-depressing drugs, endocrine hormone levels, autonomic activation, personality, mood states, environmental event-life history data, and premorbid health provided support for the idea that chronic cortical information underload promotes carcinogenesis.

Chapter 6 The Mismatch Hypothesis: Support from Studies of Non-CNS Structures

Your theory is crazy but it's not crazy enough to be true.

Niels Bohr to a young physicist

HYPOTHESIS II: ROLE OF NON-CNS MISMATCH

The following section presents evidence which suggests that optimal information load-mismatch in (generally) non-CNS somatic structures initiates carcinogenesis and determines its initial site of manifestation. While the evidence for this position is not as abundant as it is for CNS influences, there nevertheless exists a considerable body of literature suggesting that non-CNS structures have optimal ranges of information processing for organized function, and that chronic information underload and/or overload is associated with carcinogenesis.[19]

Chronic information underload or overload for a particular (generally) non-CNS somatic structure is associated with carcinogenesis in that somatic structure. The somatic structure's predisposition to carcinogenesis from either information underload or overload is associated with its relative level of development (including phylogenetic development). A relatively high level of development (a high level of growth, differentiation and organization) in a given biological structure predisposes it to carcinogenesis from information underload, whereas a minimal level of development of structure is associated with carcinogenesis from severe information overload (the latter condition effects a compensatory information underload state, the sine qua non of carcinogenesis).

EVIDENCE FOR HYPOTHESIS

Clinical, Anecdotal Observations

Many types of cancer develop at sites of chronic tissue irritation or stimulation. Cancer of the lip in an inveterate pipe smoker tends to develop where he holds his pipe (Selye, 1956).   Sir Percival Pott (Glemser, 1969: chapter 3) observed a high incidence of cancer of the scrotum in boys working as chimney sweeps, and surmised that it must have been the soot, ground into the skin of the scrotum from the boys' clothes, which later caused the malignant tumors.

Thus clinical-anecdotal impressions often suggest that chronic *overstimulation* of a particular non-CSN somatic structure is associated with the production of malignancy in that area.

Experimental Evidence

Experimental evidence points out that not only information overload but also information underload for any of several non-CNS somatic structures is associated with carcinogenesis at the site of optimal information load-mismatch.

The Cell

INFORMATION UNDERLOAD. Sanford et al (1950) found that malignant changes occurred in cultured cells that received no specific treatment.   Series of fibroblasts from adipose connective tissue or skeletal muscle of strain C3H mice were cultivated and certain groups of cultures were treated for twenty-one days with 20-methylcholanthrene in varying concentrations.   Both carcinogen-treated and untreated cultures were injected periodically into mice to test the ability of the cells to give rise to sarcomas.   Of five series of cells carried in culture more than a year in the absence of any known carcinogen, four eventually became able to give rise to sarcomas on injection; the fifth was lost before an adequate study could be made. The transformations in the four series occurred after varying periods in culture.   The limited carcinogen treatment failed to enhance the sarcoma-producing ability of the cells in the dosage range studied. Shelton et al (1963) showed that untreated cells can undergo malignant conversion in a completely isologous biological environment, demonstrating malignant transformation of normal cells in the situation of *isolation* within semipermeable capsules implanted into the peritoneal cavities of animals on the donor strain.   The sealed chambers of Millipore filter material allowed the passage of body fluids but not of cells, so that the contained normal cells were isolated from contact with other cells but were otherwise environmentally situated with access to humoral homeostatic influences. These experiments strongly suggest that the loss of cell contact, and hence the loss of information exchange between cells, is an essential component of the cancer-inducing effect.

Other instances of information underload at the cellular level effecting carcinogenesis have been reviewed by Clayson (1962).   He quotes evidence showing that the induction of tumors by the implantation of impermeable sheets of various materials, whether it be cellophane, plastics of various kinds, glass, etc., is not responsible for producing the cancer effect.   Rather, as Goldhaber (1959) has shown, it appears that it is the physical *barrier* itself that constitutes the carcinogenesis influence. By measuring the effect of pore size on the incidence of tumors following the implantation of Millipore filter material, he was able to show that if the perforations in the sheet are big enough, cell contacts can be made (information exchange obtains) and the tumors do not arise. Finally, as pointed out in Chapter 1, cancer cells are characterized by a lack of intercellular communication; they lack the junctional complexes which allow intercellular communication between adjacent normal epithelial cells (Dowben, 1971).

INFORMATION OVERLOAD.   In viral carcinogenesis, the molecular geneticist studies cancer as a problem resulting from the introduction of new genetic material or information into the cell. According to Richards (1972: 71), most tumor-producing viruses are likely to produce cancer in *newborn* animals rather than in wild animals of adult age. This fact fits in well with the writer's developmental-structural approach to carcinogenesis: minimal development of *genetic* structure implies a susceptibility to information overload. The introduction of virus (information) to a young system is more likely to result in information overload than for the more experienced organism. This is because there is relatively more information flow resulting for the less developed organism when it comes into contact with ordinary RNA and DNA viruses, which provide high levels of information flow for immature genetic structures.

In *irradiation* carcinogenesis, physical particles such as gamma and X-rays, alpha and ultraviolet particles, carry high amounts of energy and when they strike a cell a direct change occurs in the cell's chemical bonds. In addition, whole body irradiation involves a series of somatic responses such as virus release from the bone marrow, transitory depression of the immune response of the animal, and depression of defense mechanisms residing in the bone marrow and spleen (Kaplan, 1964; Kaplan, 1967). These same somatic reactions can be precipitated by information overload for the CNS, and are associated with increases in anti-inflammatory hormone activity in the body (Selye, 1956). In the terminology of the proffered conceptualization, irradiation is conceptualized as providing information; if sufficiently intense or prolonged, information-overload carcinogenesis would result, particularly in an organ or organism with relatively low development of structure.

There is considerable evidence for these predictions. In 1935, Jacob Furth showed that X-rays could induce leukemias in mice, and Goffman and Tamplin (1970a, 1970b) have reviewed the literature and suggested three generalizations concerning the induction of cancer by ionizing radiation: (1) most forms of cancer can be increased by ionizing radiation; (2) most forms of cancer show closely similar doubling doses and closely similar percentage increases in cancer mortality rate per rad of exposure; and (3) younger subjects require less radiation to increase the mortality rate by a specified fraction than do adults.

The Skin

THE STRUCTURE AND ITS INFORMATION. The skin contains melanin, a pigment-forming structure; the skin of different individuals and/or groups of individuals is characterized by different levels of development of melanin structure. Lightly pigmented individuals are conceptualized to have minimal development of structure and darkly pigmented individuals, the converse.

Melanin processes information from solar (ultraviolet) radiation. The more intense and/or the greater the exposure to such radiation, the more information is processed. The less developed the melanin structure, the more information is processed from a given temporal exposure to a given intensity of ultraviolet (solar) radiation. Thus, the hypothesis predicts that lightly pigmented individuals would be more susceptible to carcinogenesis via information overload, and darkly pigmented individuals would be more susceptible to skin cancer associated with information underload. Evidence for these predictions follows.

INFORMATION OVERLOAD. There is much literature suggesting that prolonged exposure to sunlight can result in the development of skin cancer in man (Blum, 1959; McGrady, 1964; Urbach et al, 1972). The person most likely to develop skin cancer has a light complexion, blond or red hair, and blue eyes. He or she freckles and sunburns easily and is often of Celtic ancestry (Plum, 1959; Urbach et al, 1972; Epstein, 1931; Elliot and Welton, 1946; Hall, 1950; Ten Seldam, 1963; Silverstone, 1964). Among the main arguments in favor of this suggestion are: (a) skin cancer occurs most frequently in those areas of the body which are exposed to ultraviolet radiation (Epstein, 1931; Unna, 1894; Dubrenilk, 1907; Belisario, 1959; Urbach, 1963); (b) pigmented races, who sunburn much less readily than do people with white skin, have much less skin cancer—when it does occur, it is *not* predominantly found on areas of skin exposed to solar radiation (Urbach, 1963; White et al, 1961; Fleming et al, 1975); (c) among Caucasians, there appears to be a greater prevalence of skin cancer in those who spend more time outdoors than in those who work predominantly indoors (Urbach, et al, 1972; Urbach, 1963; Gellin et al, 1966); and (d) skin cancer can be produced readily on the skin of mice and rats with repeated doses of ultraviolet radiation—the upper wavelength limit of cancer-producing radiation is about 325 nm., the same spectral range that produces sunburn in human skin (Roffo, 1939; Plum, 1959).

INFORMATION UNDERLOAD. There are reports suggesting that skin cancer often results from minimal exposure to ultraviolet solar radiation. Urbach (1963) reported that skin cancer in blacks occurs in those areas of the body which are *covered* by clothing. A similar result is described by McGrady (1964) who reported that white United States war veterans showed a high incidence of cancers of exposed areas of the skin (8.45% of all cancer) and black veterans very little (0.6%). On the other hand, the same investigator points out that the percentages for cancers of *unexposed* skin areas are reversed completely in blacks and whites—0.8% in white and 9.78% in black veterans. Fleming et al (369) studied skin cancer in black patients. They reported that 61% of squamous cell carcinomas developed in *unexposed* areas; malignant melanomas occurred most frequently on the plantar surface (sole) of the foot (76%). White et al (1961) noted the high percentage of tumors (in black patients) developing in the *covered* areas of the body. The above findings are conceptualized thus: the high level of development of melanin structure in highly pigmented individuals is associated with a relatively high need for information (ultraviolet radiation) for optimal function of that structure; the information underload obtaining upon exposure to ordinary (solar) environments for individuals with high development of melanin (structure) is carcinogenic.

The Uterine Cervix and Breast

THE UTERINE CERVIX. The cervix functions passively as a segment of the birth canal, and as a channel for the exitus of the menstrual discharge. Its primary physiological function, however, is the secretion of mucus during sexual intercourse which facilitates the transport of spermatozoa and subsequently acts as a plug to seal off the impregnated uterine cavity from the external environment. That the growth and development of the cervix parallels stimulation by estrogen (a female hormone) has been demonstated by Scheppenheim et al (1959) and Hellman et al (1954).

THE BREASTS. The breasts are modified skin gland structures which begin to show increased development during puberty with the rather sudden appearance of ovarian and female hormone activity. The functional mammary gland is one of the most highly differentiated and metabolically active organs of the body. Its principal function is lactation, which is comprised of two distinct physiological processes (Cowie, 1974), milk secretion and milk removal.[20] At the initiation of lactation, marked alterations in the general metabolism of the whole animal occur to accommodate the demands of the organ (Davis and Bauman, 1974). A redistribution of the blood supply, a marked increase in metabolic rate, and a dramatic increase in the demand for nutrients denote a few of the gross changes in the total metabolism necessary to sustain the activity of the gland. Female hormones have a consistent effect on breast development. Topical or systemic application of estrogen increases breast structure in hypogonadal or post-menopausal women and induces varying degrees of mammary development in different species. Progesterone, another female hormone, induces either duct or alveolar growth in several species; usually more rapid and extensive growth occurs after administration of both hormones than administration of either one singly. Mammary development normally goes to completion only during pregnancy and pseudo-pregnancy, periods when both estrogen and progesterone are secreted in enhanced amounts (Forbes, 1966).

INFORMATION OVERLOAD AND CERVICAL CANCER. The cervix is a relatively primitive biological structure compared to the breast. Phylogenetically, development of breast structure appears relatively late in evolution with the class mammalia, while most lower inframammalian, vertebrate animals have a uterine cervix. Ontogenetically, the same pattern of development obtains: within class mammalia, animals are born with a relatively high development of cervical structure as compared to breast structure, the latter showing comparatively more development later during puberty. Compared to the breast, the cervix (in the adult female) appears to present less differentiation of cellular structure and function than does the breast. According to the proffered hypothesis, uterine cervical cancer should obtain more often from conditions of information *overload* mismatch, since the cervix is a relatively less developed (or phylogenetically experienced) structure, and breast cancer should be associated more with information *underload* mismatch, since the breast shows a relatively high level of development of structure (there is greater redundancy and differentiation of parts).

Studies of cervical cancer generally support the hypothesis. In 1950, Gagnon (1950) demonstrated a striking lack of cancer of cervix uteri among French-Canadian nuns in the Province of Quebec. These findings were later replicated by Schomig (1953), Madigan and Vance (1957), Taylor et al (1959), Nix (1964), and Fraumeni et al (1969). Carcinoma of the cervix is much more common in women who marry or become pregnant in their teens (Christopherson and Parker, 1965), and the rate among prostitutes is extremely high (Rjel, 1953).

Cervical cancer is second in prevalence only to breast cancer among women in the United States and other Western countries. In underdeveloped countries, and indeed on a world wide basis, it is probably the most common of all cancers in adult females. Rates vary in geographic areas and even within different geographic areas of the same city (Clemmesen, 1965; Christopherson and Mendez, 1966). For example, in a metropolitan area the incidence of cervical cancer is approximately twice as high in the lowest income population compared to the highest. American black women have a higher rate of cervical carcinoma than American white women (Suss et al, 1973). All the above findings imply a positive correlation between cervical information flow rates and risk of cervical cancer. The association seems, in large part, attributable to social standing, since low social status is associated with early sexual relations, early age at marriage, frequent births (Suss et al, 1973), and incidence of venereal disease. Thus, information overload would seem to be a factor in cervical cancer. (In molecular biology, it is generally agreed that a sexually transmitted virus is associated with cervical cancer. This is compatible with mismatch theory. As described in Chapter 7, viruses may be conceptualized within an informational framework and construed to effect information overload and underload for sub-cellular structures.)

INFORMATION UNDERLOAD AND BREAST CANCER. There is much evidence suggesting that breast cancer is associated with information underload for breast structure. Stern (1844) was among the first to observe that unmarried and sterile married women have a higher breast cancer risk than do married women. Nuns have a much higher risk for breast cancer than married women (Schomig, 1950) in the older age range (Fraumeni, 1969). Prolonged nursing seems to diminish the risk of breast cancer (Richards, 1972: 126), provided the experience of lactation in a lifetime exceeds thirty-six months. In female dogs, breast cancer is most likely to appear in the most caudally situated breast or "hind-teat" (Harris, 1978), which receives less use than more rostrally situated breasts. Stated differently, shortening the length and number of periods of lactation greatly increases the risk of breast cancer (Cowdry, 1968:157). These findings suggest that failure to use the breasts for the purposes intended promotes carcinogenesis in that structure; in the language of the proffered conceptualization of carcinogenesis, long term information underload for the breast structure is carcinogenic.

Similarly, there is evidence that breast cancer can be induced by procedures which increase the level of development of breast structure, and thereby increase the information need for optimal function of breast structure and hence the probability of information underload. For example, Lacassagne (1932) was the first to show that mammary cancer can be induced (in mice) by the administration of female sex hormones (estrogens). Sinha and Dao (1972) have shown that estrogen administration enhanced mammary tumor growth. On the other hand, decreasing the level of breast structure development by certain procedures often results in the retraction of breast cancer. Beatson (1896) reported the first therapeutic ovariectomies (surgical removal of the ovaries), and other investigators found remissions in breast cancer upon the administration of male sex hormones (Richards, 1972: 108). In the language of the proffered hypothesis of carcinogenesis, breast cancer often shows regression with decreases in development of breast structure, because a lower development is associated with a lower need for information processing for organized function, and the lower need for information processing diminishes the probablity that the breast will experience information *underload* if it processes an ordinary amount of information (i.e., stimulation during sexual activity or lactation) over some time period.

The Lungs

THE STRUCTURE AND ITS INFORMATION. The lungs are elastic bag structures located in a closed cavity of the body called the thorax. The function of the lungs is to oxygenate the blood and to eliminate carbon dioxide in a controlled manner. The process of inspiring and expiring air, exchanging gases, distributing oxygen to the cells and collecting carbon dioxide from the cells is called pulmonary function. Among the basic tests of pulmonary function are those designed to determine lung volumes and capacities. For example, the total lung capacity is the amount of gas contained in the lungs at the end of a maximal inspiration. The vital capacity is the maximum volume of gas that can be expelled from the lungs by forceful effort after a maximal inspiration.

Of interest for this presentation is that these volumes and capacities generally vary with experience. Later evolving animals generally have greater volumes and capacities than animals evolving earlier since the lung evolved relatively late in evolution. Similarly, ontogenetically older lungs (but excluding gerontological populations) have greater volumes and capacities than younger ones. Short term increments in lung experience or development, for example, as would obtain for individuals participating in a rigorous body-conditioning program, would be associated with relatively greater lung volumes and capacities compared to the pre-conditioning program baseline when the lungs were less experienced or developed. Volumes and capacities are about 20% to 25% less in females than in males of most species, including the human species.

Information theory suggests that information for the lung varies with the number of alternative elements in the atmosphere breathed. Generally, the constituents of atmospheric air are oxygen, nitrogen, water, and rare gases such as krypton, argon, etc. Polluted air contains these gases plus organic particulate matter such as polynuclear, aromatic hydrocarbons, the latter being shown to be carcinogenic to several animal tissues (Wynder and Hoffman, 1967; Hoffman and Wynder, 1968). Tobacco smoke contains tar and a significant quantity of alkylated 4- and 5-ring aromatic hydrocarbons which seem to have strong carcinogenic activity (Hoffman and Wynder, 1968; Wynder and Hoffman, 1972).[21] Thus polluted air and tobacco smoke differ from unpolluted air in the number of contained alternative elements, polluted air and tobacco smoke containing all of the elements of unpolluted air plus additional elements. In this sense, the amount of information (defined as $\log_2$ of the number of alternative elements) processed by the lungs upon exposure to tobacco smoke and polluted air is enhanced relative to the amount of information processed by the same lungs upon exposure to unpolluted air.

INFORMATION OVERLOAD AND LUNG CANCER. There is abundant evidence supporting the view that information overload for the lung associated with cigarettes and with breathing polluted air is often carcinogenic. This evidence, in large part, has been derived by epidemiological methods involving statistical studies of masses of populations. In general, most studies suggest that the more heavily one smokes, the longer one smokes, and the earlier one starts smoking the higher the probability that one will develop lung cancer (Richards, 1972; Hammond, 1966; Wynder and Hoffman, 1967). There seems to be a general association between information overload (from tobacco smoke) and carcinogenesis. There is also epidemiological evidence indicating that in the moderately polluted greater Los Angeles area, younger individuals develop a significantly higher incidence of lung cancer (Sullivan, 1973) than older individuals. According to the hypothesis, this obtains because an organ (organism) having minimal development of lung structure is more likely to experience information-overload upon exposure to a polluted atmospheric environment than is the organ (organism) with relatively greater development of structure.

Most forms of lung cancer in mature adults who smoke cigarettes are conceptualized to occur when the amount of information provided by the cigarette smoking *greatly* exceeds the information processing capacities of certain tobacco-sensitive structures in lung (mainly epidermoid-squamous cells). The *extreme* information overload is posited to effect a switching-in of a compensatory, protective information-reducing response by these overstimulated structures. The result is an information *underload* condition which subsequently signals the need for novelty, i.e. cancer.

INFORMATION UNDERLOAD AND LUNG CANCER. There are some data suggesting that lung cancer also may develop in response to information underload for the lung. According to Richards (1972), 10% of lung cancer victims never have smoked and 95% of heavy cigarette smokers never contract cancer. The writer's hypothesis would predict that the 10% who have never smoked may have a high level of development of lung structure such that their lungs have been chronically understimulated by an insufficiently complex atmosphere. It is conceivable that some of the 95% of heavy cigarette smokers who never contract cancer might have developed cancer had they not smoked; heavy cigarette smoking might be adaptive for individuals having a high level of development of lung structure, since the higher the level of structural development, the higher the information need for organized function of the structure. There exist scattered reports (Doll and Hill, 1959; Schwartz et al, 1961), indicating that among heavy smokers, non-inhalers may have the greater risk for lung cancer.

Sex differences in lung cancer may also be explained within this theoretical framework. Incidence of lung cancer is comparatively rare among women, the ratio (circa 1970) being six to one higher for men (Richards, 1972: 129). The suggestion here is that this disparate ratio obtains, in part, because the average male lung is more likely to experience either chronic information overload or information underload relative to the typical female lung. Information overload is more likely for some males because many more males than females work in jobs which involve their being exposed to extremely information-rich atmospheres, and more men than women smoke cigarettes (although this is changing rapidly as more women enter the work force and as society's attitudes toward acceptable feminine behavior become more flexible). On the other hand, information underload is also more likely for some males since their relatively greater development of lung structure implies that a greater proportion of them will experience information underload on exposure to *ordinary* nonpolluted environments. The average male lung, owing to its relatively high development of lung structure relative to the typical female lung (i.e., as indexed by greater lung volumes and vital capacity; a greater size implies greater "redundancy" and a greater buffering capacity to environmental change or information), and hence having a relatively high need for lungular information for optimal organization of function, will be more likely to experience information underload on exposure to *ordinary* unpolluted atmospheric environments.[22]

The Colon

THE STRUCTURE AND ITS INFORMATION. The colon, a muscular tube, is part of the gastrointestinal tract. Its primary functions are the temporary harboring of the waste products of digestion, the mixing and drying of the stool, and the delivery of the stool to the rectum for evacuation. These functions require a variety of periodic propulsive but coordinated movements called laxation. Information for the colon might vary with the amount and/or rate of stool passed per unit of time. Foods containing a significantly larger amount of indigestible material (fiber) pass through the intestinal tract very quickly compared to foods containing lesser roughage. High fiber foods would provide the colon a high rate of information processing relative to low roughage foods. Observations of patients suffering from chronic constipation showed that compared with normal subjects, they had a greater capacity to break down the crude fiber in certain fruits and vegetables in the alimentary tract, with resultant failure to secure satisfactory laxation in the colon. Constipation thus represents relative information underload for the colon since a minimal amount and/or rate of stool (information) is being passed per unit of time.

INFORMATION UNDERLOAD AND COLON CANCER. There is evidence suggesting that dietary habits markedly influence colonic cancer. The lowest incidence of colon cancer is found in countries in which the typical diet is high in fiber content; the highest incidence is found in Western parts of the world (cancer of the colon and rectum killed 47,000 Americans in 1973, ranking the disorder second to lung cancer in deaths). The typical Western diet which leans heavily on refined sugar and flour, and is low in fiber content, is associated with decreased information processing for the colon.

A low incidence of large bowel cancer has been found throughout the continent of Africa in the indigenous population.   The incidence rates in immigrant groups tend to approach those of their new (usually Western) environments (Stein, 1974).   Burkitt (1971) has assumed that initially the black slaves had as little bowel cancer as Africans do now, and he considers the rise in the incidence of bowel cancer to be the result of the adoption by American blacks of the food habits of the Caucasian population.   Lawrence (1936) claims that many years ago when much more maize was eaten by American blacks, especially by those living in the South, the incidence of bowel cancer was slightly more than half that of the Caucasians.   This difference has almost disappeared (Doll, 399) with the blacks' adoption of the Caucasians' food habits.

The Stomach

The hypothesis predicts that eating a diet consisting of mainly one class of food (e.g., carbohydrates) would result in information under-load for the stomach and hence predispose towards the development of stomach cancer.   Glemzer (1969:   311-312) and Modan et al (1974) suggest that stomach cancer is often associated with a diet consisting chiefly of carbohydrates.[23]

Other Cancers

The proffered conceptualization of carcinogenesis in other somatic structures of the body would be consistent with the model described for skin, lung, genital-breast, colon, and stomach cancer. That is, non-CNS structures such as the pancreas, liver, bone marrow, bone have some optimal range of information processing (where information is defined relative to each structure's function and level of develop-ment), and chronic information underload and/or overload for each structure is associated with carcinogenesis.

SUMMARY

In summary, there is considerable evidence suggesting that chronic information underload or overload in non-CNS somatic structures is associated with initiation of carcinogenesis in the structure experi-encing the optimal information load-mismatch.   Evidence presented vis-à-vis carcinogenesis at the level of the cell, the skin, the breast and uterine cervix, the lung, the colon, and other somatic sites, strongly supports the hypothesis that a somatic stucture's predisposi-tion to develop cancer from either information underload or informa-tion overload is associated with the specific structure's relative level of development.   In general, the described findings support the hypothesis that a relatively high level of development in a given non-CNS biological structure predisposes the structure to carcinogenesis from information underload, whereas a minimal level of development predisposes the structure to carcinogenesis from severe information overload (and subsequent compensatory isolation).

Summary of Mismatch Hypothesis

The major focus of Chapters 4 and 5 was to suggest a possible central nervous system (CNS) modulating component in carcinogenesis. Literature review suggested that the CNS exerts a generalized non-specific *modulating* (promoting or inhibiting) effect on carcinogenesis. Chronic information underload (CNS depression, the experience of boredom) for the central processor of the brain was posited to *promote*, while chronic information overload (CNS activation, the experience of excitement) was posited to *retard* the development of most types of carcinogenesis in mature, experienced organisms.

It was suggested that most types of spontaneous, rapidly-spreading cancers in adult organisms are *promoted* by information underload (boredom) experienced by the brain over some relatively prolonged temporal interval. When the information deficit reaches some critical value, the brain sends a nonspecific signal to most somatic structure sites (usually non-CNS structures) indicating the need for novelty or information; carcinogenesis is the body's mode of providing "information-novelty" which is subsequently fed back to the brain and which attempts to rectify the relative information underload signaled by the brain. In the later stages, the develpment of cancer is also associated with an increase in the disorganization (entropy) of the organismic system. The increased disorganization is associated with an increase in the amount of information processed from the environment. In the late terminal stages the cancer may also provide information to the CNS in the form of pain by invading or pressing on surrounding tissues which are supplied with nerves, or by leading to pressure on nerves themselves. The pain is then fed back to the brain to help rectify the brain-signaled information deficit. Conversely, chronic information *overload* for the brain is posited to result in a compensatory response by the brain to *decrease* the probability of novelty, i.e. cancer, obtaining in most somatic structure sites.

On the other hand, *extreme* levels (chronicity, intensity) of information underload/overload (boredom, excitation) were seen to be associated with "paradoxical" cancer-retarding/promoting effects, respectively. These effects are apparently associated with the brain's effecting compensatory, homostatic changes in its own rate and/or amount of information processing. This apparently occurs in order to provide some more optimal range of information processing needed for the brain's own organized function. For example, when the brain (central processor) experiences *extreme* information underload and/or extreme boredom, it often effects a compensatory information-inundating, physiologically-activating state (i.e., hallucinations and/or increased motor activity) which feeds back information and subsequently effects a paradoxical inhibition of carcinogenesis. Similarly, under conditions of *extreme* information inundation and/or extreme excitation, the brain "switches in" a compensatory, protective, information reducing, low-activation state which was observed to be associated with a paradoxical promotion of many cancers.

Chapter 6 has suggested possible ramifications of the developmental-structural approach to cancer *initiation* and pointed out that a comprehensive model of cancer etiology need consider not only psychosomatic aspects at the CNS level, but also possible *psychosomatic* aspects in non-CNS somatic structures. Literature review pointed to the possibility of an *initiating* psychosomatic component in (generally) non-CNS structures which is specific in effect and which dictate the site of initiation of carcinogenesis. Thus it was argued that some varieties of neoplastic disease are initiated by chronic information underload (and/or severe overload), which subsequently effects underload) at specific non-CNS somatic structure sites. Information for various non-CNS structures was defined as "novelty" and/or stimulation. For example, a varied diet or a diet containing foods of high information content (e.g. proteins) was argued to provide more information for the stomach than a diet composed exclusively of carbohydrates. Information for the breast was argued to vary with the number of lactation periods and/or the degree of stimulation during sexual activity. Information for the immunological system was posited to vary with the novelty of circulating antigens, viruses, bacteria, etc. For cellular and sub-cellular structures (DNA, RNA, etc.) information was conceptualized to vary with the novelty of interacting stimuli (or products of stimuli) such as viruses, chemicals, irradiation, etc.

Carcinogenesis is thus considered an information control mechanism by which chronically isolated structures attempt to effect a more optimal rate of information flow for themselves when orthodox information control mechanisms have proven inadequate in rectifying the information deficit. Initially, carcinogenesis provides isolated structures short-term homeostatic increments in rate of information flow. This is accomplished principally by the disorganizing effects of the metastasizing cancer cell on previously organized (automatized) infra-structure function. With continuing mestastasis, however carcinogenesis becomes heterostatic not only for infra-structures but also for the isolated structure and its supra-structures (the organism, the family, etc.).

Literature review suggested possible biochemical and physiological mechanisms whereby chronic information underload for the CNS may promote carcinogenesis. Several studies pointed to an association of low rates of information flow in the CNS, mediated by parasympathetic autonomic activity, with increases in mitotic rate, DNA synthesis, and growth hormone release. These findings suggest that chronic isolation from information (phenomenologically: boredom) may promote carcinogenesis by enhancing the numerical proliferation of cells, the genetic material of which has been altered by direct contact with carcinogenic agents, or by increasing the number of spontaneously occurring "copying errors" during DNA replication, thus increasing the probability of the genesis of new mutant cancer cells.

Chapter 7 The Mismatch Hypothesis: Explanatory Utility, Predictions, and Implications for Preventive Medicine

> *Those who dream by night in the dusty recesses of their minds wake in the day to find that it was vanity; but the dreamers of the day are dangerous men, for they may act their dreams with open eyes, to make it possible.*

> T. E. Lawrence
> *From the suppressed/introductory chapter of* **Seven Pillars of Wisdom**

EXPLANATORY UTILITY OF THE HYPOTHESIS

Environmental Variables: Radiation, Viruses, Chemicals, and Psychophysiological Stress

As pointed out earlier, the information load-mismatch hypothesis may have considerable explanatory utility vis-à-vis the effects of environmental variables. Radiation, chemicals, viruses and psychophysiological stress may be re-defined in information (and/or stimulation) terms. For example, a sensory environment providing sensory stimuli of variable duration and intensity is conceptualized to provide the brain more information than an environment in which intensity and duration are less variable (except when the former condition provides *extreme* sensory flow, in which case compensatory information-reducing mechanisms are called into play). Muhlbock's (1950) finding that mice develop spontaneous mammary tumors significantly earlier if the animals are raised in isolation might be explained in an information underload framework. That is, understimulated cortical structures promote novelty at the cellular level i.e. carcinogenesis. Findings that various types of clinical and experimental cancer often are significantly retarded by infections, intoxications and various drugs can also be handled by mismatch theory. These nonspecific stressors increase information flow for the cortex to high levels; cortical structures then act to minimize the probability of additional information flow at the cellular level by minimizing the probability of mutations (new cancer cells).

Mismatch theory posits that all biological structures process information from their environments. Any structure may experience a mismatch between its optimal information load and the amount of information provided by its environment. Mismatch theory applied to data on lung, gastrointestinal, and skin structures was described in Chapter 6. Sanford et al's (1950) and Shelton et al's (1963) findings of malignant changes in isolated cells can be handled within an information underload framework. Mismatch theory applied to viruses and various chemicals follows later in this chapter.

Geography-cancer interrelation may also be conceptualized in the mismatch framework. Different geographical areas will vary with respect to informational environments, primarily because of cultural and naturalistic factors. For example, the decrease in stomach cancer in Japanese who immigrate to the U.S. might be explained as due to rectification by the U.S. diet of an information-poor (for the stomach) Japanese diet. That is, Modan et al (1941) found that stomach cancer is often associated with a diet consisting chiefly of carbohydrates. Carbohydrates have been found to have a much lower stimulating effect on gastric acid secretion than proteins (Saint-Hilaire et al, 1960). Since the Japanese, in general, will consume a more varied diet (and one higher in protein and fat) in the U.S. than in Japan, it is possible that the traditional Japanese diet is not optimally informative for stomach structures. The resulting information underload, carcinogenic for the stomach, is rectified by the relatively information-rich diet obtainable in the U.S.

Biological Variables

Sub-cellular and cellular structures

The hypothesis has possible applications to sub-cellular mechanisms in carcinogenesis. Nucleic acids are complex molecules representing the simplest manifestation of life since they are the first compounds in the hierarchy of molecules capable of reproducing themselves and of transmitting their characteristics to the progeny. One type called deoxyribonucleic acid (DNA) is found in the nuclei of cells and is the material of which genes are composed. Another type, ribonucleic acid (RNA), is found in the cytoplasm of the cell. The DNA is the repository of all the information necessary for the formation of protein and for the reproduction of the cell. The genetic message of the nucleus can be carried from the nucleus to the cytoplasm on a strand of RNA called "messenger" RNA. This substance wraps itself around the ribosomes in the cytoplasm and gives them the information necessary for identical genetic replication (Richards, 1972).

The four bases of DNA, namely guanine (G), cytosine (C), adenine (A) and thymine (T), form the language of life; all that can be passed on about life in the recesses of our cells requires only the code G-C-A-T. The sequence of any three of the four letters determines the specificity of a given amino acid (i.e., role and duty). The same is true of any information essential to the life and reproduction of the cell. Once in a great while a different grouping of the bases occurs, altering the composition of the DNA. The resulting mutation is of great interest. In cancer, the cell is a changed cell which does not behave like a normal cell and thus may be the outcome of a mutation. Cancer may be the result of a direct spontaneous mutation within the genome (or entire genetic information) of the cellular DNA, or cancer may result from carcinogenic agents in the external environment influencing the cell. The origin of malignant cancer and its vagaries is apparently wrapped up in these genomal and extragenomal changes in the normal cell (Richards, 1972).[24]

The four different bases (adenine, cytosine, guanine, and thymine) are structures which process information from an environment comprised of other bases, sugars, phosphates, and other cellular structures. Information transfer, for example, presumably occurs between the pairs of bases, held together by hydrogen bonds across each strand of the helix. As in other biological structures, there presumably exists an optimal range of information processing for each base. For example, it is a fact that the amount of adenine in the double-stranded helix is always equal to the amount of thymine and the amount of guanine is always equal to the amount of cytosine in the linked-based pairs (Richards, 1972). Optimal information load-mismatch for a given base would be effected by a change in a base of the normal DNA template; i.e., either an alteration, substitution or deletion, such that the structure of the affected base is changed in a way that it or its linked base is likely to experience optimal information load-mismatch. For example, in viral DNA incorporation the subsequent synthesis of viral-dictated chemical processes may effect information overload; on the other hand, base deletion by mutation—spontaneous or otherwise—may effect a loss of genetic information and hence effect information underload.

Chemical carcinogens interact with a wide variety of cellular macromolecules (cf. Ruddon, 1981, pp. 213-227, for an excellent review). Apparently, the interactions usually involve alkylation of nucleophilic (electron-rich) groups on nucleic acids or proteins with electrophilic (electron-seeking) groups of the carcinogen. Covalent binding of various carcinogens to proteins in target tissue has been shown. Both the carcinogenic nitrosamines and aromatic amines have been shown to interact with nuclear histones, indicating a possible direct effect on chromatin-regulatory proteins. The role of these carcinogen-protein conjugates in carcinogenesis has not been elucidated. One hypothesis is that the carcinogen binding proteins may act as receptors for carcinogens to permit the translocation of the carcinogen to the cell nucleus; another idea is that the proteins promote the interaction of the carcinogen with chromatin or DNA in the nucleus or even with the various types of cellular RNA. Mismatch theory predicts that the attachment of carcinogens to bases in DNA and RNA in some way effects a condition of either information underload or *severe* information overload (which subsequently effects information underload), and that information underload subsequently signals the need for novelty—mutation—in the hereditary material of the cell. For example, attachment of chemical carcinogens to bases in RNA and/or DNA may prevent normal base-pairing during messenger RNA translation and/or DNA replication, and thus lead to the biosynthesis of novel, but faulty, proteins (i.e cancer) via optimal information-load mismatch mechanisms (deletion, substitution, etc. of bases).

Ruddon (1981) suggests that a number of points made about chemical carcinogenesis are also true for radiation-induced carcinogenesis. Both X-rays and ultraviolet radiation produce damage to DNA, which induces DNA repair processes, some of which are error prone and may lead to mutations. Various theoretical conceptualizations of carcinogenesis from a molecular biology viewpoint (viral, chemical, irradiation) exist. In time, molecular biological research will demonstrate which hypotheses and speculations have more credibility and validity.

The major point of this section is to suggest that the optimal information-load mismatch notion suggested by the author's relatively molar and holistic approach may have application at the molecular level. That is, in molecular biology, one moves from the particular to the general, via the construction of larger concepts from an understanding of molecular mechanisms. The systems orientation, on the other hand, proceeds from the general to the particular; i.e., the construction of "the part" from an understanding of relatively molar mechanisms. In the phraseology of the legendary Hermes Trismegistos: "As above, so below." (The present author does not have the requisite backround to assess the validity of the mismatch hypothesis for molecular phenomena; this endeavor could be more efficiently accomplished by individuals working in the field of molecular biology.)

Phylogeny

The finding of an enhanced proclivity for the development of genuine malignancies with increasing phylogenetic development can be handled by mismatch theory. At the core of phylogenetic development is an enhanced memory store and/or capacity. The development of a larger memory store minimizes the amount of information processing (and/or CNS activation) the organism extracts on exposure to everyday environments, because much of the information is already in the organism's memory store. The result is a diminution of experiences of mismatch between expected and contacted stimulation, and thus a relative diminution of the orienting response and/or CNS activation obtains on a "characterologic" basis. Compared to organisms with minimal phylogenetic development, those with relatively greater development are conceptualized to be in a chronic state of relative functional information underload and/or low physiological activation. The findings of an enhanced probability to develop genuine malignancies with increasing phylogenetic experience thus coincides with the optimal information load-mismatch hypothesis which posits that chronic information underload and/or CNS depression enhances the probability of most forms of carcinogenesis.

Ontogeny

As described earlier, cancer generally appears in the post-reproductive period of life, between the ages of forty-five and sixty-five. Findings in the ontogeny of cancer support the hypothesis in the same manner described for the phylogeny of cancer. Increased experience in the adult is associated with an augmented memory or model of the environment. The more comprehensive model of the environment minimizes the probability of surprisal or information processing from ordinary environments, because much of this information is already in the adult's memory, and a minimizing of mismatches between expected and environmental stimulation occurs. The result is a reduction of orienting responses and concomitant physiological deactivation in most environmental-organism interactions relative to that obtaining for the child or less experienced organism.

Evidence from developmental studies of sensory information processing capacities and physiological activation was presented earlier. In the main, these studies point out that increasing age is associated with higher sensory thresholds in the major sensory modalities (vision, audition, pain, etc.) and lowered cortical activation (EEG slowing).[25] There is a suggestion from studies of cognitive function in gerentological populations (Owens, 1957; Eisdorfer, 1963; Schaie and Strother, 1964; Eichorn, 1973) that the relatively large decrement in sensory information processing in old age is not accompanied by as large a decrement in cognitive information processing capacity. Decrements in physical capacity, as defined by tests of physical strength and endurance, more or less parallel decrements in sensory information processing capacity with age; i.e., lung, cardiovascular and muscle capacities diminish significantly with increasing age. These findings suggest that the CNS of older adults may be construed to experience a higher degree of functional sensory information underload than younger adults, since the former's CNS structure is relatively intact (shows a high degree of development and organization) and thus still needs a relatively high level of information for organized function. But the usual channels for supplying much of the information—sensory information channels, including exercise-related sensory information channels—are capable of providing only a limited amount of the optimal range needed for organized brain function. It is posited here that the typical older cortex experiences considerable information underload relative to the relatively younger cortex. Unable to rely on the usual sensory information processing channels for much of its own input, it resorts to the creation of somatic information via carcinogenesis as a last resort to effect some optimal level of information processing for its own organized function.

Sex hormones

The explanatory utility of the model for cancer of the uterus and breast has been described in great detail in an earlier section and will not be reviewed here. The hypothesis also applies to other structures influenced by sex hormones. In 1939, Huggins (cf. Richards, 1972: 107) obtained remission of cancer of the prostate in man by removal of the testicles, the main sorce of male sex hormones (androgens) controlling the activity and growth of the prostate gland. In the mid-1940s, Dodds et al (cf. Richards, 1972: 107) discovered methods for preparing active synthetic estrogens (female hormones) which could be administered orally; Huggins showed that remissions could be obtained with hormone therapy rather than by castration. These findings can be conceptualized along the same information load-mismatch lines discussed for breast cancer.

Genetic predisposition and personality factors

Literature reviewed earlier pointed out that hereditary influences exist which predispose some individuals to cancer. Since hereditary factors presumably operate in the development of somatic structure, hereditary predispositions of some individuals, families and groups of individuals (races) to develop cancer would be explained in part on hereditary factors in the development of both CNS and non-CNS somatic structures.

   Similarly, since certain dimensions of personality (activity level, aggressiveness) are to some extent influenced by genetic factors and are presumably associated with development of brain structure, the information load-mismatch hypothesis can be used to explain literature findings vis-à-vis the "cancer personality". For example, development of brain structure is associated with low physiological arousal [26] and a subsequent need to actively engage the environment (hyperactivity, high energy level), excessive ego development and control (impairment of discharge of affect, inadequate outlets for instinctive drives, etc.), and a tendency to psychological depression or melancholia when the environment fails to provide sufficent information and stimulation.

Points of Overlap with Other Hypotheses

The information load-mismatch hypothesis of carcinogenesis has some points of overlap with other proffered hypotheses. It has commonality with Virchow's chronic irritation hypothesis in positing that chronic over-stimulation of tissue is carcinogenic. However, it goes beyond that hypothesis in defining more precisely the nature of a stimulus or irritation for a receptor structure, in differentiating the concept of physical injury stress from psychophysiological stimulation, and in dealing with the complex problem of stimulation or information for epithelial as well as mesenchymal tissue. Moreover, the proffered hypothesis can account for the finding that the absence of irritation (information underload) enhances the probability of carcinogenesis.

The information load-mismatch hypothesis and the immunological deficiency hypothesis [27] have points of overlap and congruence. There is evidence that in order for cancer to occur and persist, there must be a failure of the immunological process (Southam et al, 1957).[28] Selye (1956) and others (Petrovoskii, 1961; Meerloo and Zeckel, 1952; Fessel, 1962; Fessel and Forsyth, 1963; Korneva and Khai, 1963; Korneva, 1967; Rasmussen et al, 1957; Marsch et al, 1963) have demonstrated that variations in levels of CNS activation and/or information processing (as effected by lesion, brain stimulation and stress conditions) are associated with changes in immunological competence. In general, these studies suggest that information overload stress is associated with a diminution of immunological competence, and information underload stress is associated with an enhancement of immunological competence, and that these relationships are reversed at the extremes of information overload and underload stress. Wistar and Hildeman (1960) subjected mice to long-term avoidance conditioning with electric shock and observed subsequent skin transplantation immunity. The stress condition could be argued to have produced an information overload condition, since the electric shock was very predictably delivered. Strict alteration of current was delivered to each half of the wired floor of the shuttlebox at six minute intervals and the mice were reported to have learned very quickly how to avoid the shocking current. (Animals were subjected to this stress six hours per day, six days per week for two weeks before grafting, and again after grafting until homograft rejection was complete). Vessey (1964) observed that information underload (isolation in separate one-gallon jars) is associated with significantly higher levels of circulating antibodies than is information overload. (In each of three experiments five to six mice were placed in a metal can three feet in diameter for only four hours per day for the duration of the experiment). Solomon (1969) found that moderate (but not severe) over-crowding stress significantly reduced primary and secondary antibody response in rats to flagellin, a potent bacterial antigen.

There is evidence for paradoxical responses of the immunological system to extreme level information load-mismatch conditions (Weltman et al, 1968; Hatch et al, 1963; Monjan and Collector, 1977). Weltman et al (1968) matched seventy female albino mice by body weight and divided the group into isolated and control groups. All isolated mice were housed singly in stainless steel cages. The number of control mice per cage was limited to populations of two. All mice were allowed to eat *ad libitum,* and were allowed to drink tap water freely via stainless steel sipper tubes. All animals received equivalent degrees of handling; day-night noise levels and room temperature were controlled during the twenty-six week experimental observation period. Tail blood specimens were taken at four, eight, twelve, twenty-two and twenty-four weeks for total leukocyte counts and at weeks twenty-two and twenty-four for eosinophil counts. The major finding was that white blood cell counts were higher in isolates than in controls during the fourth week of the observation period, but as the isolation period continued, the total leukocyte count in the isolates showed marked *decreases* while the controls showed minimal change from the fourth week, so that at the twenty-second and twenty-four weeks of observation, the isolates showed significantly *lower* white blood cell counts (both total leukocyte and eosinophil counts) than the non-isolated controls. Thus, moderate-to-high level information underload (here defined as four weeks of isolation) is associated with an enhancement of development of antibody structure, but extreme level information underload (twenty-second to twenty-fourth week of isolation) is observed to be associated with a paradoxical response (i.e., decrease in development of structure) of the immunological system. Hatch et al (1963) reports that short-term (up to ten days) information-underload stressed (isolated) rats show smaller adrenals as compared with animals kept in groups of two or more; in contrast, long-term isolation (longer than a month) usually is associated with just the opposite effect; i.e., a tendency to larger adrenals.

Since decreases in total leukocyte and eosinophil cells have been associated with increased adrenocortical function (Gordon, 1955; Harkonen and Knotinnen, 1958), and increased adrenocortical function is generally associated with increasing size of the adrenals, the Hatch et al data suggest that short-term isolation, interpreted here to produce a moderate information underload stress condition, is associated with *increases* in total leukocyte and eosinophil cells, i.e., enhanced immunological capacity. As the isolation becomes more severe (a condition of extreme high level information underload is produced), a compensatory CNS excitatory state is "switched in" by the CNS to help rectify the experienced information deprivation. Increased adrenocortical function would accompany the compensatory CNS excitatory state and would be associated with increasing size of the adrenals and decreases in total leucocyte and eosinophil cell count.

Monjan and Collector (1977), working on the information overload side of stress, also report paradoxical responses of the immunological system to a stressor condition of relatively short versus relatively long term duration. Male mice (seven to twelve weeks old) of the AKR or C57/Bl$_6$ strains were subjected to broad band noise at about 100 db daily for five seconds every minute during a one or three hour period around midnight, at the height of the animal activity cycle. Unstimulated controls were exposed only to the sound activity of the animal room. Clear demonstration of stress-induced modulation of immune function was found: short-term (roughly first ten days) exposure to the sound stressor clearly depressed the leukocyte-mediated cytotoxic response, while enhancement occurred with longer exposures (up to thirty-nine days). Assays of plasma cortisol in similarly stressed C57/Bl$_6$ mice showed an increase in the circulating levels of this adrenal corticosteroid corresponding to the depression of the immunological function, but not apparently associated with enhancement of immunological function.

The above findings are consistent with the general notions

outlined earlier vis-à-vis pro- and anti-inflammatory hormone-CNS activation (and/or information processing) interrelations and the proffered mismatch hypothesis of carcinogenesis. That is, CNS depression and/or information underload is associated with the building-up of relatively high level immunological structure as indexed by a relatively high level of circulating white blood cells, is mediated by the dominance of pro-inflammatory over anti-inflammatory adrenal cortex hormone activity, and generally acts to promote carcinogenesis. On the other hand, CNS activation and/or information overload is associated with the breaking down of immunological structure as indexed by a relatively low level of circulating antibodies, is mediated by dominance of anti-inflammatory endocrinological hormones and generally acts to inhibit most forms of carcinogenesis in adults.

Extreme information underload and/or CNS depression is associated with collapse of immunological structure as indexed by a relatively low level of circulating antibodies, is mediated by relative dominance of anti- over pro-inflammatory adrenocortical hormone activity, and is often observed to effect a paradoxical inhibition of most forms of adulthood carcinogenesis since the CNS switches in a compensatory excitatory, information-augmenting state of consciousness to help compensate for the extreme cortical information underload experienced.

Extreme information overload and/or CNS activation would be associated with a building-up of immunological structure as indexed by a relatively high level of circulating antibodies, would be mediated by dominance of pro- over anti-inflammatory adrenocortical hormones, and would effect a paradoxical promotion of carcinogenesis associated with the CNS's switching in of a compensatory inhibitory, information-reducing state of consciousness to help compensate for the extreme information overload experienced by the CNS.

The conclusion that most forms of carcinogenesis in adults are promoted and/or enhanced by environmental-CNS structure interactions associated with pro-inflammatory adrenocortical hormone dominance is congruent with reviewed findings indicating that (1) pro-inflammatory adrenal hormones resemble in many of their actions the tranquilizing agents (chlorpromazine and reserpine), while anti-inflammatory hormones mimic in many ways CNS stimulating drugs such as the amphetamines; and (2) it is possible to inhibit the growth of many cancers by anti-inflammatory hormone treatment (Selye, 1956; Kavetskii, 1960; Trainin, 1963). Viewed in another way, pro-inflammatory hormones promote anabolic processes which conserve energy and which repair and build-up somatic structures. The often-observed effectiveness of anti-inflammatory hormones on certain types of carcinogenesis would be explained thus: anabolic dominance characterizes the pre-morbid state of the majority of adult individuals who later develop cancer; anti-inflammatory hormone administration helps to restore the anabolism-catabolism balance needed for organized adaptive function. On the other hand, the above considerations suggest that a minority of adulthood cancers (certain leukemias, perhaps) possibly associated with extreme information overload would be ameliorated by moderate doses of pro-inflammatory hormones, since this would bring CNS activation within the moderate-to-high level range, a condition inhibitory to most forms of adulthood carcinogenesis.

IMPLICATIONS OF THE MISMATCH HYPOTHESIS FOR FUTURE RESEARCH

General Implications

According to the hypothesis, the probability of carcinogenesis is minimized when CNS and non-CNS structures experience information load-match from the environment, so that levels and/or amounts of information processing for the structures fall within some optimal range needed for organized function of the structures. For example, the hypothesis would predict that skin carcinoma (melanoma) would be minimized in the following way: a light complexioned individual (low development of melanin structure) would take care to avoid too much exposure to sunlight, and a dark complexioned individual (high development of melanin structure) would take care to expose himself to sufficient sunlight to ensure that his relatively high need for solar radiation is met. Both individuals would also take care to provide their brains with moderate-to-high levels/amounts of information-novelty in their day-to-day living environments.

On the other hand, the probability of carcinogenesis is maximized when a given non-CNS somatic epithelial structure(s) experiences sufficiently intense and/or protracted environmental information load-mismatch, so that levels and/or amounts of information processing for the structure(s) fall outside some optimal range needed for organized function; and when the brain experiences either information underload mismatch or extremely high level information overload, the latter switching in a compensatory inhibitory state of information underload. It is predicted that skin cancer would have a relatively high probability of developing in a light complexioned individual who exposes himself to too much sunlight (information overload for the melanin in his skin) and whose brain has been experiencing either information underload (lack of stimulation, boredom, etc.), or extremely high level information overload; and in a dark complexioned individual who fails to expose himself to enough sunlight (information underload for his melanin structure) and whose brain has been experiencing either information underload or extremely high level information overload.

Boredom as a Phenomenological Precursor

The mismatch hypothesis posits that information underload (boredom) promotes most cancers of epithelial tissue. Several environmental conditions and situations generally evocative of the experience of boredom are known to be associated with the promotion of carcinogenesis. Loss of a spouse or an important interpersonal relationship and (social) isolation has been found to precede the development of many tumors (LeShan, 1961; LeShan, 1962; LeShan, 1959). Since most adults depend a great deal on their spouses for a significant part of their day-to-day stimulation, the loss of such an important source of stimulation could be associated with the production of information underload and the experience of boredom.

The hypothesis thus predicts that relatively long-term isolation (social and/or sensory), accompanied by the experience of boredom and/or CNS depression, is an antecedent of carcinogenesis. Other environmental conditions and/or situations associated with this experience would be predicted to be associated with carcinogenesis: conditions fostering a relative restriction of mobility and movement, such as breaking a leg or being unable to travel to new environments due to lack of funds, being unable to take vacations (which de-automatize perception), would be predicted to antedate the development of cancers. If REMS during REM sleep can be assumed to represent quanta of sensory information (as suggested by my SCIP hypothesis of REM sleep function (de la Peña, 1971), then chronic sleep deprivation or voluntary sleep curtailment (associated with job, general living requirements) may promote carcinogenesis. That is, although the brain sleeps more efficiently with deprivation of sleep, (i.e. more compensatory deep and REM sleep during shortened sleep periods) delta sleep is compensated more efficiently than REM sleep in total sleep deprivation. The result is a brain deprived of some quantity of endogenously-generated sensory information or stimulation; this information-lack would be associated with information underload (phenomenologically: depression, fatigue, boredom) for the brain which could be rectified to some extent by information-augmenting activities, e.g. delusions, hallucinations, behavioral hyperactivity, cancer, etc. (cf. de la Pena, 1971). Moreover, since deep sleep and low levels of waking physiological activation associated with depression, fatigue, boredom (i.e. low blood pressure, heart rate, muscle tension) are associated with growth hormone release, and carcinogenesis is characterized by abnormal growth of cells, there is congruence in the hypothesis.[29]

The hypothesis predicts that the predisposition for many forms of carcinogenesis may be indexed by various sleep-dream characteristics. In the pre-morbid stage, predisposition to carcinogenesis is posited to be indexed by relatively short latencies to the first REM sleep period, relatively high phasic REM densities during REM sleep periods, excessive daytime sleepiness and/or insomnia (associated with boredom), and relatively poor dream recall compared to age-sex norms. All of the above sleep characteristics are found in conditions characterized by low waking sensory information flow (e.g. narcolepsy, endogenous depression, insomnia associated with boredom, some forms of sleep apnea, old age, etc.). As the cancer develops and begins to metastasize, the increments in cancer-produced sensory information flow (from pain, infectious processes, disorganization of organ functions, etc.) results in relative normalization of the sleep-dream behaviors. However, in the fully malignant stage, sleep-dream characteristics would show a dramatic turn-about (long latencies to REM sleep, decreased density of REMs, good dream recall) reflecting a response to the abnormally increased levels of waking sensory information flow and generalized systemic entropy.

Psychophysiological Predispositions

The hypothesis predicts that given chronic exposure to ordinary, sensory environments, certain individuals with certain nervous system characteristics should show an enhanced proclivity to develop cancer. For example, an individual with a very high level of development of CNS structure would process a modicum of information from an *ordinary* sensory environment and thus experience a high degree of boredom and/or information underload predisposing to carcinogenesis. Or similarly, an individual with "constitutional" relatively high sensory thresholds (which would effectively serve as a stimulus barrier) would be predisposed to develop carcinogenesis, as would an individual with low levels of physiological activation[30] (low levels of blood pressure, heart rate, muscle tension, high basal skin resistance, etc.), and manifesting behavioral hyperactivity (or hypoactivity).

Polednak (1976) provides some data which suggest support for these notions. He conducted a survey of over 8,000 college men. Among major athletes (which he defined as having lettered in various college sports) an excess risk of cancer of the prostate and digestive tract, excluding the colon, was found. This data corroborated other data from several studies indicating that major athletes die significantly more often from cancer than non athletes. Polednak concluded that levels of fitness characteristic of competitive athletics are not synonymous with optimum health and might actually be destructive.

Since athletes generally have lower levels of physiological activation (lower heart rate, blood pressure, etc.) and higher sensory thresholds associated with physical conditioning (and perhaps with constitutional factors), it is possible to view the athlete as an individual having a very low degree of biological noise and/or a very high degree of automatization in most somatic structures. The enhanced automatization of physical function is associated with information underload upon engaging in *ordinary* physical activity (walking, talking, sitting, etc). Optimal information flow for highly developed physical structures occurs during enhanced physical activity. Forced inactivity, as from incapacitating injury, or the curtailment of activity accompanying the aging process and its sequelae (rheumatism, obesity, cardiovascular problems, etc.), would be conceptualized to produce information underload stress in individuals (such as athletes) who have highly developed physical structures. Since the greater the level of development of structure(s), the greater the need for stimulation for optimal function, athletes would be particularly disposed to experience information underload when physical activity is curtailed. (Many instances of forced inactivity, as from incapacitating injuries, can be found in the biographies of world class athletes who subsequently developed cancer).

Predictions of the Hypothesis: Biochemical and Endocrinological Aspects

The hypothesis predicts that the majority of adulthood cancer patients should show relatively low levels of adrenocortical steroid output (e.g., urine and plasma corticosterone) and/or low levels of circulating norepinephrine in the *premorbid* state compared to individuals who do not later develop cancer.   With the onset of carcinogenesis, these relationships should reverse, since in many instances the cancer process apparently is attempting to reverse or compensate for the prior organismic condition of information underload. Findings of high levels of free fatty acids (FFA) and ACTH in plasma of cancer patients (Cardon and Mueller, 1965, Ruddon, 1981), where FFA levels and ACTH are considered a rough index of sympathetic nervous system activity and/or excitatory cortical processes, would be explained along these lines. That is, it is posited that premorbid levels of FFA and ACTH in individuals later developing cancer would be relatively *low* compared to individuals who do not later develop cancer. Subsequent development of cancer would be associated with a compensatory rise in FFA and ACTH levels in plasma, mirroring the compensatory information-load enhancing effect of cancer.

The hypothesis also predicts an association between serum cholesterol and predisposition to develop cancer.   That is, high levels of information flow (stress, anxiety) associated with uncertain, unpredictable environments generally increase serum cholesterol levels. Boredom and/or low information flow levels are theoretically associated with low serum cholesterol levels. Several studies (cf. *Consumer Reports*, May 1981, p. 260) including one conducted recently by the National Heart, Lung and Blood Institute, have found a significant association between low serum cholesterol and increased cancer mortality, particularly colon cancer. Whether low serum cholesterol is a correlate of the posited etiological factor in carcinogenesis (low levels of information flow, boredom, dominance of anabolic versus catabolic processes, etc.), or a *secondary* compensatory effect in response to the carcinogenic process remains to be determined by future research.

Findings pointing out the procoagulant activity of cancer cells (Donati, Davidson, and Garattini, 1981; Gralnick, 1981) are also consistent with the mismatch hypothesis. Mismatch theory predicts that individuals who develop cancer of epithelial tissue will have low premorbid levels of procoagulant activity.   This is because most cancer prone individuals are posited to have an excessively strong parasympathetic autonomic nervous system and/or a weak sympathetic system as a consequence or correlate of the development of cognitive structure. Development of cancer cells i.e., novelty introduction at the cellular level, would have an activating effect on the sympathetic autonomic nervous system, particularly in the later stages when pain is experienced.

Since activity of the sympathetic branch of the autonomic nervous system increases the coagulation of blood and the parasympathetic branch retards clotting ability, the procoagulant activity of the sympathetic branch of the autonomic system in the cancer process is posited to represent a compensatory response to excessive parasympathetic dominance in the pre-morbid state (cf. also Robinson 1980, for discussion of work on tumors which secrete catecholamines).

The Need for Systematic Research on Unconventional Therapies

The mismatch hypothesis suggests that the scientific establishment give more serious consideration to the various unconventional forms of cancer treatment. That is, the hypothesis predicts that agents or chemicals that increase CNS activation and/or which increase the information processing rate in the CNS should protect against many forms of adulthood cancer (mainly the epithelial variety), since the posited etiological condition of information underload and/or low CNS activation is rectified by these treatments.

Dietary Approaches

Diets and/or vitamin therapies employing megavitamin doses of vitamins C, A, and the Bs seem especially worthy of more study, since these vitamins are known to affect amounts of excitatory neurotransmitters such as epinephrine and norepinephrine in the CNS. Epinephrine and norepinephrine, for example, are produced from tyrosine under the influence of vitamin C. Vitamin C also protects against oxidation of the two neurotransmitters (Kutsky, 1973) and hence would effect increased levels of circulating, excitatory, information-augmenting neurotransmitters in the CNS. Studies are emerging which describe the efficacy of vitamin A in the treatment of lung cancer (Saffioti et al, 1967; Cone and Nettesheim, 1973; Bjelke, 1975) and epithelial tumors (Bollag, 1970).

In *Cancer and Vitamin C* (Cameron and Pauling, 1979), a great deal of evidence is reviewed which supports the notion that regular high intakes of vitamin C is helpful both in the prevention and treatment of cancer. Cameron (1966) had previously pointed out that the resistance of the normal tissues surrounding a malignant tumor to infiltration by that tumor would be augmented if the strength of the intercellular cement that binds the cells of the normal tissues could be increased. He noted that this intercellular cement contains very long molecular chains, called glycosaminoglycans, that give it strength, and it also contains fibrils of the protein collagen, which further strengthen the cement. Cameron had also pointed out that some, and perhaps all malignant tumors liberate the enzymes hyaluronidase and collagenase, which cause the glycosaminoglycans and collagen fibrils respectively to be cut into smaller molecules, thus weakening the intercellular cement.

In 1971, Cameron and Rotman suggested that an increased concentration of vitamin C in the body would help stimulate the normal cells to produce increased amounts of the substance hyaluronidase inhibitor, which would combine with the enzyme hyaluronidase, liberated by the malignant tumor, and prevent it from attacking the intercellular cement. At about the same time, Pauling pointed out that it is known that vitamin C is required for the synthesis of collagen; increasing the intake of this vitamin would effect the production of more collagen fibril, further strengthening the intercellular cement. (Despite the rationales, Pauling and his colleagues have been unsuccessful in attracting any significant funding support from the National Cancer Institute and the American Cancer Society.)

The use of Laetrile or amygdalin in cancer deserves more study. Amygdalin is a complex subtance which occurs in seeds of *Rosaceœ*, especially almonds and apricot seeds, from which it can be obtained by extraction with alcohol. Almonds and apricots are rich sources of vitamins A and B. Practitioners of the Laetrile treatment of cancer often prescribe vitamin C, in addition, usually in megavitamin doses (Cameron and Pauling, 1979); put the patient on a vegetarian diet, a regime similar to Gerson's (1958); and add digestive enzymes and large amounts of vitamin A and other vitamins and minerals. More research is needed to test out those agents of the total treatment which often appear, at least anecdotally, to help cancer patients.

Immunological Approaches

Numerous animal and human experimental studies have demonstrated that stress, psychological depression, and other psychological factors compromise an organism's capacity to prevent the onset of cancer or limit its spread (Klein, 1966). Interaction between the host's neurophysiological and immunological systems is pointed out to be the key element in such phenomena (cf. Achterberg et al, 1976 for an excellent annotated bibliography of this research). However, the data are very disparate; some studies find that stress is immunosuppressive, while others find that stress enhances immunosuppressiveness (cf. Kaliss, 1965). Much more systematic research is needed in this area; special attention needs to be paid to the nature of stress (information overload versus underload), duration-intensity of stressor conditions, level of development of host's neurophysiological and immunological systems, etc. Only when all of these variables are considered is there a chance that a semblance of order will appear in the literature.

Imagery Approaches

Upon extensive research into the imagery of cancer patients during states of deep relaxation, Achterberg and Lawlis (1977) formulated a test (termed Image-Ca) which takes the subjective reports of patients and scores them in a manner which can be objectively reported and considered.   In their study, data from 126 cancer patients were collected over a one-and-a-half year period, and patients were administered an extensive battery of psychodiagnostic tests along with the Image-Ca, and hematological analyses. Their research allowed conclusions that blood chemistries reflect ongoing or concurrent disease state, that there is a statistical relationship between blood chemistries and psychological variables and that psychological factors are predictive of subsequent disease status. Further, data from follow-up study indicated that psychological factors were better predictors of patient outcome than hematological analyses.

Encouraged by their early results, Achterberg and Lawlis developed Image-Ca to provide clinicians with a means of assessing the role that patients play in their own treatment. Patients participated in a relaxation procedure and were asked to focus on their own subjective images of their cancer cells. Subsequently they were asked to draw the images they had seen. Structured interviews were conducted; the researchers recognized fourteen scorable dimensions which were amenable to standardization and qualification.   Results of their research are detailed in the diagnostic manual *Imagery of Cancer: An Evaluation Tool for the Process of Disease* (1978).   The researchers noted that there were some common elements in the imagery indicative of a positive and negative prognosis.   Images such as "white knights," "Vikings," "large, powerful animals, especially dogs and bears" which were visualized to aggressively attack the cancer cells were associated with the best prognosis.   Less vivid, less dynamic imagery was associated with a less favorable prognosis.

In the conceptual framework of the present writer's developmental-structural approach, the Achterberg-Lawlis technique of utilizing imagery techniques, may be conceptualized to induce an increase in the amount of sensory information flow and/or level of CNS activation relative to pre-morbid levels. Perhaps the technique is effective to the extent that cancer patients can utilize this technique of sensory information (imagery) augmentation to rectify the posited low levels of sensory information flow which the mismatch hypothesis deems a critical etiological element in carcinogenesis.   Future research should strive for classification of the role of imagery, which could be varied with respect to dimensions such as vividness, dynamic character, color complexity, etc., in the treatment of cancer. Comparisons with externally generated sensory information conditions would be of interest.

Holistic Physical Approaches

Another line of research, while molecular in approach, emphasizes the holistic approach on optimum states of function rather than the medical establisment's emphasis on pathology. In his book *Electronic Biology and Cancer* (1976), Szent-Györgyi points out:

Cancer research has greatly been retarded by our asking why cancer grows, instead of asking what keeps a normal cell from growing . . . . Cancer was looked upon as a hostile intruder which had to be eliminated. It might be looked upon also as a cell in trouble, which needs help to return to normal.

Szent-Györgyi advances a hypothesis of cancer based upon molecular interactions prior to oxygen, the β state. He maintains the problem resides in a "lack of oxygen" which has been found to "induce a malignant transformation in tissue cultures. It is easy to believe that a lack of O_2, which induces changes in other factors, will eventually take the cells back from the oxidative β state to the fermentative α state." When a cancer cell falls into the α state, a state of high fermentation, the problem is not its rate of proliferation but that it does not stop dividing when no further replication is required. Szent-Györgyi's hypothesis is complex and has yet to be adequately tested. However, his thesis is compatible with the mismatch hypothesis, in that the low rates of information flow in biological structures, hypothesized to be cancer promoting, are associated with low levels of oxygen saturation in these structures; further his approach is innovative in that it posits optimum levels of function (information processing) in cells as the critical factor which should be promoted in order to help cells maintain accurate replication. Research along these lines is clearly worthy of funding support, but to date has not attracted funding from national agencies and foundations. In need of testing is the idea that deprivation of oxygen is the critical element in inducing cancer. That is, the work of Shelton and her colleagues (1963) and Sanford et al (1950) suggests that it is deprivation of *information* per se that is carcinogenic.

IMPLICATIONS FOR THE TREATMENT OF CARCINOGENESIS

General Implications

The mismatch hypothesis has clear implications for the treatment and/or prevention of carcinogenesis. The practice of isolating cancer patients in wards, particularly in the early stages and/or initiation phase of the process when it is not yet irreversible, possibly exacerbates the development of some cancers, because such isolation is associated with the information underload condition which apparently promotes many cancers. The hypothesis implies that cancer can be inhibited in the early phases of the process by environmental conditions which provide information and/or novelty for the patient. Also implied is the potential therapeutic utility of certain psychotomimetic drugs which enhance cortical physiological activation and/or sensory information processing (moderate-to-high doses of amphetamines,

LSD, marijuana, etc.) in the treatment of the majority of cancers of adulthood. In the posited minority of cases in which carcinogenesis is associated with extreme chronic information overload and/or physiological activation, administration of moderate-to-high doses of tranquilizing agents and/or parasympathomimetic drugs (phenothiazines, reserpine, etc.) might be of therapeutic value.

One of the most revolutionary implications for preventive cancer medicine suggested by mismatch theory is the notion that the propensity for carcinogenesis is minimized when there is a close match between a structure's information organizing capacity and the amount of information afforded by the structure's environment. The capacity of the brain to process information, "model" the stimulus events and/or configurations, and habituate to the environmental constancies can in some instances (as when neurometric techniques are available) be directly measured. However, it is unlikely that direct measures of cortical and other structural information organizing capacities would be readily available for a majority of individuals. Indirect and approximate measures of cortical development could be inferred from information about intellectual and educational achievements (year of school completed, scholastic honors, degrees obtained, inventions, etc). Indirect measures of lung and cardiovascular development could be inferred from behavioral and self-spouse reports of aspects of physical activity such as endurance and participation in athletic endeavors demanding strenuous exertion (e.g., swimming, long distance running, basketball). A rough measure of breast development would be afforded by brassiere cup size, using overall body weight as a correction factor. On the other hand, level of development of cardiovascular status could be directly assessed by levels of such variables as heart rate, blood pressure, vital capacity, total lung capacity, etc., during resting and stressful conditions; high levels of development would be indexed by a relatively quick return (relative to age-sex norms) to baseline following stressful conditions, by high values for vital capacity, and low values for heart rate and blood pressure.

Along with assessments of level of structural development, the patient's "environment" could also be studied with an eye towards rating its information content. For example, the information flow for the breast over a given temporal interval would be determined by the frequency and duration of periods of lactation and sexual activity during that interval. Level of information processing for the lungs would be indexed by aspects of atmospheric informational complexity such as number of cigarettes smoked per day, degree of atmospheric pollution of general and work environment, frequency and intensity-duration of physical exercise, etc. Level of information processing for the cortex could be assessed by self and/or significant others' ratings of general sensation seeking, boredom thresholds, proclivity to psychological depression and loneliness, etc.

After assessment of structural developmental levels and levels of information flow for the different biological structures, the relative degree of match or mismatch between structural needs and environmental characteristics could be inferred. Relatively high levels of mismatch for any structure would indicate the utility of intervention in the patient's life, either via biological or environmental manipulations, so as to minimize the probability of mismatch.

The Central Role of Consciousness and Experience in Preventive Medicine

In the proffered framework, "experiential" activity plays the central role in preventive medical practice. That is, biological and psychological order (health) is preserved to the extent that a structure is able to realize some optimal range/rate of information processing. The higher the level of development of structure, i.e., the greater the amount of potential mismatch in the direction of information underload, the greater the information flow needed from the environment or from endogenously-produced activity. There exist myriad avenues of stimulation for the relatively automatized structure. The automatized structure may increase its rate of information flow by engaging the environment more vigorously (e.g., increasing one's general level of physical,[31] intellectual, or emotional activity). However, since all parts of the organism do not experience the same degree of underload, it is likely that an excessively automatized brain may initiate far more activity (information processing) than is optimal for other less developed (and hence less automatized) parts of the system (muscles, joints, etc.). The result is health in one part of the system (the brain) at the expense of disease in other parts of the system (e.g., the sequelæ of over-exercising). Preventive medicine practice would assess optimal ranges and/or rates of information flow for all levels of structure in the hierarchy of structures which comprise the body.

In this conceptual framework, "interesting" experiential activities are the best preventive medicine for boredom, the prevalent problem of our times (Steinberg, 1978; Seidenberg, 1973; Ramey, 1974; Csikszentmihalyi, 1975). The problem is that with increasing experience or age, the average Western adult finds less and less of the world interesting because, in a sense, most of the information is already in the mind. The current practice of forced retirement at a given age is not healthy because the developed brain needs information to keep it working in a healthy, organized manner. It is a commonplace observation that many individuals develop illness and die soon after retirement.

One primary goal of present day psychology should therefore be to teach individuals that consciousness is not necessarily a passive phenomenon; rather, it is a process or variable over which the individual has some degree of control. The significance of attentional habits in the control of consciousness was suggested by William James (1890: 424) who wrote that "each of us literally chooses, by his way of attending to things, what sort of universe he shall appear to himself to inhabit." Jean Hamilton (Holcomb) (1977, 1981) has more recently reviewed the growing body of literature which supports the idea that deployment of attentional controls regulates experiential and/or mood states (also see Csikszentmihalyi, 1978).

The implication of this large body of literature is that one can develop attentional strategies to help realize a match between one's information organizing capacities (needs) and the amount of information provided by the environment. That is, one can learn to see "the universe in a grain of sand," either by exposure to didactically presented material or by learning certain psychophysiological procedures (meditation, autohypnosis, biofeedback-assisted cognitive-behavioral training, etc.) which teach the individual self-control of information processing through attentional techniques. One can learn to unlearn automatic ways of processing information, and hence learn strategies for minimizing boredom and/or information underload. Similarly, one can learn how to automatize attention should one encounter too much information in one's environment.[32]

A second revolutionary implication of the mismatch hypothesis pertains to levels of structure within the hierarchy of structures in nature. That is, mismatch is posited to obtain not only for small structures such as single cells, but also for larger structures such as the brain and liver as well as macroscopic structural units such as family and state.

In the proffered theoretical framework, the more developed the structure, the greater the information processing needs for organized function of the structural unit.[33] The increasing violence, the ascendance of sporting events and entertainment, all with their inherent uncertainty and excitement, no doubt provide a certain amount of de-automatization (increased information flow) for increasingly developed automatized group and individual "minds." Short-lived peace treaties, never-ending wars and conflagrations, particularly among developed, industrialized nations, suggest the possibility of highly automatized individual and group "minds" which avoid the boredom of peaceful co-existence in their constantly seeking dangerous and uncertain confrontations with each other.

The implications for nations and societies is clear: in order to minimize potentially lethal conflicts, encourage more opportunities in the arts and sciences, as well as in the entertainment and sports fields. Arts and sciences (cf. Prentsky, 1979), entertainment and sports all provide channels wherein individuals, societies, and nations can rectify, to some extent, the low intensity of consciousness which is a natural consequence of development and the evolutionary process. Thus we might in the future not only consider talking about individual health and our personal doctors, but also about societal health (sociologists) and societal doctors (sociopathologists) or therapists.

IMPLICATIONS FOR THE THEORY OF CARCINOGENESIS

Carcinogenesis as a Form of Creativity

The information load-mismatch hypothesis posits that carcinogenesis, in many instances, is a "sub-structure" somatic process which attempts to compensate for information load-mismatch experienced by the CNS and/or other super-structures. This view of the etiology of carcinogenesis is clearly at odds with that of the molecular approach which emphasizes exogenous causation by viruses, chemicals, etc. Literature review and the proffered conceptual synthesis are more in agreement with the conclusions of the relatively molar, dynamic systems approach to cancer which has crystallized in the writing of Bahnson and Bahnson (1964: 844). They write:

> Although, to the social evaluative self, tumors may appear to be disgusting, dangerous, and foreign, on the deepest and most archaic level of primary process fantasy the creation of a tumor may be as important and meaningful to the cancer patient as is the creation of a symphony to the musician or a plastic form to the sculptor. It seems to us that we must try to understand the formation of tumors as a determined psychobiological reaction rather than as an intrusion of a puzzling foreign matter. The revolutionary contemporary development in psychophysiology, with new emphasis on the neuroendocrinological and hormonal mechanisms which mediate between experience and biological process, most likely soon will make it feasible to study the biochemical and physiological processes which intervene between the narcissistic and regressive discharge of psychological drive and the creation or facilitation of neoplasm.

Bennette (1969:361) also has expressed a systems viewpoint of carcinogenesis which is in agreement with the proffered hypothesis. Upon reviewing evidence for the role of psychic and cellular aspects of isolation and identity impairment in carcinogenesis, he concludes:

> We could develop the idea that invasive cancer results from an internalization of disturbances of identity and communication that cannot find psychic expression because of the strength of well-differentiated psychic controlling functions, that is, a strongly developed or hypertrophied ego, coupled with inadequate bodily homeostatic control; on the other hand, where the ego and other psychic controls are poorly developed, but there is a competent

bodily homeostasis, a similar disturbance of deep identity would lead to psychotic regression. On this basis, malignant diseases and regressive psychoses could be seen as alternative biographical expressions of illness proneness, in the sense that they are comparable but differently balanced modes of evolution of the same underlying pathology, a pathology of alienation.

A New Bent to the Term "Psychosomatic"

The term *psychosomatic* is the mind-body problem[34] expressed in medical terms (Bahnson, 1974). Heretofore, the term has referred exclusively to CNS and/or brain influences on non-CNS somatic, physical processes. For example, business worries, presumably mediated through the CNS, often are observed to cause ulcers, a non-CNS somatic physical process. The proffered conceptual approach to carcinogenesis suggests that the term psychosomatic can be generalized from CNS processes to non-CNS somatic structures as well. That is, evidence described earlier for information load-mismatch for non-CNS somatic structure sites implies that information load-mismatch can be recognized or experienced by biological structures or units of organizations at *each* level in the hierarchy of levels of organization which comprise an organism (Koestler, 1967), and that the information load-mismatch may be signalled to sub-supra and same-level structures. Thus carcinogenesis induced by information underload at one level of structural organization can be rectified to some extent by introducing the appropriate compensatory information-load into another level of the whole system. For example, skin cancer, according to the proffered conceptualization of carcinogenesis, is caused by information load-mismatch at the level of the melanin (structure) in the skin and by information load-mismatch in the CNS. However, skin cancer can be influenced by introducing information to the immunological system in the form of BCG, an exotic stimulus to the system. Apparently, there is some supra-level system or supra-unit of structure which is sensitive to "total organism" amount of information processing and which acts to control some optimal amount of information processing for organized function of the whole organism.

The foregoing considerations imply that each unit of organization in the organism has some optimal range of information processing for organized function. Optimal information load-mismatches at each level unit of organization are communicated to supra-, sub- and same-level structures, signaling the need for compensatory amounts of information processing to help keep the level range of information processing within the limits necessary for the survival of each unit.[35]

Chapter **8** Extensions of Mismatch Theory to a Broad Range of Health Phenomena

The early phases of a science require the power of a broad, sweeping intellect that has a certain disregard for the formalisms and pedantic, creeping construction of the ultimate scientific edifice. Perhaps what is essential is a fountain of sensible, if vague, ideas and orienting attitudes—correct in their broadest sweep if not in their precise predictions.

Jack P. Hailman
Science, 168, 701 (1970)

INTRODUCTION

This chapter reviews the considerable literature in support of a radically new conceptualization of health and disease. The major contention is that many psychological, behavioral and somatic phenomena which the medical establishment labels "disorder" and "death," are part and parcel of the evolutionary process. Disorder and death are considered manifestations of covert compensatory homeostatic mechanisms employed by excessively automatized micro and macro-units in nature (cells, brain, nature) to effect a higher, more optimal rate of information flow for their own organized function and integrity. That is, excessive automatization of information processing, brought about by increments in experience and/or repeated exposure to stimulus environments, effects a decrease in the amount/rate of information flow for psychobiological structures to *sub-optimal* levels for organized function of the structures. Excessively automatized structures (cells, brains, nature) modulate information flow to higher, more optimal levels for organized function by promoting perceptions and behaviors (including illness and death) which serve a de-automatizing role.

HEALTH PHENOMENA ASSOCIATED WITH INCREMENTS IN EXPERIENCE:

Somatic Phenomena

A wide variety of so-called "somatic" phenomena, traditionally labeled disorders, apparently are associated with increments in cognitive structure and concomitant automatization of cortical attentional processes. Their expression appears to be modulated by short-term decreases in information flow (as during isolation or sleep) for the brain. In less severe or less chronic instances, expression of the phenomena may play a homeostatic function in rectifying information-underload mismatch for the brain, in that excessively low levels of information flow for the brain can be compensated for by endogenous somatic mechanisms, thus mitigating the extent to which the organism must actively engage a potentially hostile environment in order to realize optimal information flow for the brain.

Asthma

In asthma, the bronchioles of the lung become excessively constricted, thus impeding airflow in and out of the lungs. Asthma rarely becomes severe enough to cause serious anoxia, but it often may cause such extreme respiratory effort that severe dyspnea results. The treatment of choice is a variety of CNS stimulating drugs (theophylline, epinephrine, etc.) which relax the bronchiolar musculature. Observations (Kinsman et al, 1974) and studies (Spector et al, 1976) suggest that asthma is associated with excessive activity of the parasympathetic autonomic nervous system in a parasympathetically-tuned (dominant) nervous system (Gellhorn and Kiely, 1973).

In both phylogeny and ontogeny, the parasympathetic branch of the autonomic nervous system develops later than the sympathetic branch, is more highly differentiated with respect to function, and is thought to be associated with energy conservation (anabolism), protein synthesis, and the development of inhibitory cortical processes considered necessary for rational, logical thought processes and sleep. Gellhorn and Kiely (1973) have taken the parasympathetic-sympathetic autonomic activation concept a step further and have introduced the trophotropic (rest-inducing) and ergotropic (work-inducing) systems. They write (:236-237):

> Procedures leading to increased sympathetic discharges are accompanied by cerebral excitation, increased activity and tone of the striated muscles, and behavioral arousal. Conversely, increased parasympathetic activity is associated with a lessening of somatic action: the EEG shows sleep-like potentials; the muscle tone is lessened, and drowsiness, sleep, or coma supervenes. In the former case we

speak of activation of the E-system (ergo-tropic), in the latter of the T-system (trophotropic).

The two systems are further characterized by mutually reciprocal relations and tonic activity. With increasing excitation of the E-system there is an increasing degree of inhibition of the T-system and vice versa: increasing stimulation of the posterior hypothalamus, the reticular formation, or the sciatic nerve produces growing pupillary dilation even after sympathetic denervation of the eye and adrenodemedullation. Tonic activity and reciprocity lead to release phenomena. Transection of the brain stem between anterior and posterior hypothalamus releases the E-system, producing greatly enhanced general activity and loss of sleep. Conversely, lesions in the posterior hypothalamus cause a release of the T-system and sleep or coma results. In both cases the T-E balance has been altered.

Since reciprocal innervation tends to intensify the effects of E-excitation, the question arises as to whether homeostatic forces are mobilized under these circumstances. This is indeed the case. As in spinal reflexes, rebound phenomena occur following E-T excitation. Thus a hypothalamically induced sharp rise in blood pressure and heart rate is followed by a sudden decrease of these reactions immediately after stimulation. The rebound effects are not confined to the autonomic nervous system but appear also in somatic reactions and behavior. Repeated arousal, for instance, is followed by slowed, synchronized EEG potentials and behavioral sleep.

Of relevance here is that asthma appears relatively late in phylogeny with the development of a centralized nervous system and, in general, also appears late in ontogeny (although a small percentage of children manifest it early in life).

Excessive parasympathetic activity generally follows periods of increased sympathetic autonomic nervous system activity as a rebound phenomenon, e.g., following periods of exercise, anger. Parasympathetic activation is also high during deep sleep and REM sleep. Parasympathetic activation effects constriction, while sympathetic activity produces dilation of the bronchioles. That there is parasympathetic dominance in asthma is also suggested by the treatment of choice (CNS stimulating drugs) and by observations that asthma attacks usually abate when the individual experiences a *novel* environment, e.g., childhood asthma often abates when an asthmatic child spends a few days away from the habituated-to home environment, as in visiting a friend in a new unfamiliar environment. Conversely, asthma attacks are frequent during sleep, when parasympathetic activation is high.

These considerations suggest that asthma may at times provide compensatory augmentation of sensory information (associated with the symptoms of the asthmatic attack) to rectify aberrantly low levels of sensory information flow for the cortex, i.e., the attacks serve a de-automatizing function and serve to keep cortical information processing rate within certain critical limits for maintenance of structure and function. In this view, asthma, at least the less severe and/or acute variety, may have an adaptive function in the survival of the individual and species. That is, without the alerting, deautomatizing, information augmenting effect of asthma, the aberrantly low levels of CNS activation might necessitate the performance of behaviors (information-seeking, risk-taking, impulsive behavior, etc.) in order to keep CNS activation within critical limits necessary for integrity of CNS structures, or conversely, might be associated with such a low level of information flow (e.g. during sleep) that the individual might be relatively more vulnerable to anoxia and/or a host of environmental dangers (predators, natural disasters, etc.).

Hypoglycemia

Hypoglycemics commonly display chronic fatigue, apathy and anxious depression. The characteristic biochemical correlate is a relatively flat glucose tolerance curve with a tendency to steepness in decline in blood glucose two to three hours after the administration of concentrated glucose.

Experimental animal studies have shown that the neural control of blood sugar depends upon balance between the sympathetico-adrenal and vago-insulin systems (Gellhorn, 1943). Physiological and pharmacological excitation of the right vagus nerve, which innervates the pancreatic islets of Langerhans, leads to a fall in blood sugar. Vagotomy increases the ergotropically mediated elevation of blood sugar in response to stress (Gellhorn and Loufbourrow, 1963). On the other hand, adrenodemedullation results in a fall in blood sugar in stressed animals. Findings that electrical stimulation of the anterior hypothalamus produces a fall, and of the posterior hypothalamus a rise, in blood sugar (Ban et al, 1956) point out that parasympathetic or trophotropic dominance is a primary factor in hypoglycemia.

Theoretically, one would expect that the effects of such overactivity of the vago-insulin system might be eliminated by altering autonomic balance toward the ergotropic or sympathetic side. The finding that atropine reduces, and that vagotomy eliminates, the flattening of the glucose tolerance curve characteristic of the condition supports this interpretation.

Finally, it is known that hypoglycemia appears relatively late in evolution with the development of a centralized nervous system. In ontogeny, hypoglycemia is, for the most part, a phenomenon appearing late in life, although newborns are also likely to show a relatively high incidence (Barness et al, 1974). Presumably this occurs early in life before the maturation of sensory systems and information processing capacities, i.e., during a period of time when lack of maturation of structures acts as a passive barrier to reception of sensory information (cf. Genzmer, 1882; Pratt, 1946; Vinogradova, 1961; Benjamin, 1965).

I suggest that hypoglycemia is a sequela of evolution and excessive automatization of attentional processes (boredom). The excessively automatized (bored) brain rectifies its own sub-optimal rate of information flow to higher levels by initiation of an increased sympathetic autonomic nervous system discharge which is accompanied by the experience of anxiety. Theoretically, any psychological state characterized by automatization of attentional processes (depression, helplessness, NREM sleep, etc.) would be expected to induce hypoglycemia; if severe enough, the brain would rectify the low blood sugar by switching in compensatory homeostatic processes which raise the blood sugar dramatically (i.e., transient or chronic diabetes).

Duodenal Ulcer

A relatively high rate of gastric acid secretion is a concomitant of this disorder (Mirsky, 1958). The formation of the ulcer is assumed to depend on the corrosive effect of hydrochloric acid. Secretion of acid is excessive during the night in most duodenal ulcer patients as a result of the physiological shift toward parasympathetic dominance (Gellhorn and Kiely, 1973). Vagotomy reduces nocturnal acid secretion to a level equaling only one-fourth to one-third of that in the normal non-ulcer population (Dragstedt, 1956). During non-REM sleep, the posterior hypothalamus is reciprocally inhibited, as indexed by lowered blood pressure, pulse rate, body temperature, etc.; the effect is a further increase in the nocturnal vagal influence upon gastric secretion. Studies by Storer (1959) suggest that the anterior hypothalamus, which largely controls parasympathetic reactions to emotional cues, may be in a state of heightened responsivity in the ulcer patient; this conclusion is supported by observations that such patients are additionally noted to show other signs of parasympathetic dominance such as bradycardia, relatively low blood pressure levels, postural hypotension, and a tendency to easy fatigability.

Study of the gastric secretory responses of Brady's "executive" monkeys (1958, 1962) point out the "rebound" feature of gastric acid secretion in ulcer. During the time animals are engaged in shock-avoidance activity, gastric acidity is only slightly increased. Significant increments began *at the end* of the avoidance sessions and reached a peak several hours later while the animal was *resting* and away from stimulation. Thus, a maladaptive rebound of trophotropic activation in response to ergotropic excitation apparently obtains in trophotropically-tuned individuals.

Migraine

In migraine, cerebral vessels dilate excessively and press on surrounding nerves, causing pain. Cerebral vasodilation is associated with excessive parasympathetic rebound in a trophotropically tuned nervous system. That is, cerebral vasoconstriction occurs during periods of excitement and with increases in activation of the sympathetic nervous system. After the "stress" is over, there is an excessive parasympathetic response associated with levels of CNS activation dropping below pre-stress "baselines." Thus, migraine typically occurs during periods of time when information load from the environment drops to relative low levels, as during the night, during weekends, on holidays, etc. The pain of migraine may be conceptualized to rectify the abnormally low levels of information flow in the CNS associated with excessive rebound of parasympathetic activity in a parasympathetically-dominant system following a period of heightened sympathetic activity.

In agreement with the above notions, pharmacological regimens in migraine utilize treatments (caffeine, cafergot) which are stimulating to the CNS. Moreover, migraine is a phenomenon appearing relatively late in phylogeny and ontogeny, i.e., with development of cognitive (cortical) structure and the resultant high level of parasympathetic activity associated with automatization of attentional processes. Finally, data from personality studies indicates that migraineurs generally are characterized as cerebral, obsessive-compulsive, and perfectionistic, all of which suggest relatively high levels of cognitive development.

Chronic Pain Syndromes

So called psychogenic pain syndromes (chronic low back pain, tension headache, etc.) are observed to occur in older, sedentary and bored, depressed individuals as compared to younger, active and relatively happy people. In all former instances, there is apparently a relatively low level of CNS activation and/or information flow. The understimulated brain is ostensibly attempting to rectify information underload by inducing endogenous information in somesthetic and/or proprioceptive channels. The success of recent treatment suggested by the gate control theory of pain (e.g., electrostimulation of sensory nerves) suggests support for the notion that the brain attempts to rectify information underload in some patients via initiation of endogenous pain-associated sensory stimulation.

Obesity

The low level of sensory information flow (i.e., dominance of trophotropic processes) that attends states of boredom and depression, as well as the aging process, would be predicted to be associated with some forms of obesity. That is, trophotropic dominance is associated with conservation of energy (anabolism) which results in the building up of a surfeit of energy and/or "matter." The excess avoirdupois, in turn, effects an augmentation of external stimuli (attention of others to unusual shape), as well as effecting de-automatization of attentional processes for the obese person, i.e., the person becomes more aware of himself through the change of body form, proprioceptive cues, changes in dress and activity, etc. The de-automatization of attentional processes helps to rectify the primary problem of excessive automatization of attentional processes in bored, depressed individuals. That obesity is generally a phenomenon of middle and old age, when automatization of attention is theoretically at its zenith, dovetails nicely with the proffered hypothesis.

High Blood Pressure

High blood pressure is a disorder appearing relatively late in phylogeny and ontogeny. In my experience, it sometimes develops in individuals who previously had relatively low levels of blood pressure. For example, I have observed this phenomenon in looking through the medical records and charts of individuals who have developed narcolepsy, sleep apnea, and other conditions associated with excessive daytime sleepiness and/or low levels of CNS activation. That is, early in life blood pressure is relatively low. At some point in ontogeny, usually coincident with clinical manifestation of the sleep disorder, blood pressure increases to above-norm levels. Apparently, the brain may be attempting to rectify the low level of information flow by increasing the blood pressure, since increases in blood pressure are generally accompanied by decreases in sensory thresholds, the latter permitting increases in the amount of *sensory* information flow for the brain, and decreases in *cognitive-ideational* information flow. In this view, high blood pressure is often a secondary compensatory response by the brain to rectify excessive automatization of attentional and physiological processes.

This view of the significance of blood pressure elevation is clearly at odds with the current establishment viewpoint but is in clear agreement with recent ideas and findings in contemporary psychophysiology. That is, an acute rise of blood pressure is recorded by baroreceptors in the aortic arch of the heart. Baroreceptor stimulation, in turn, lowers blood pressure by reflex actions on the heart and blood vessels (Koch, 1932; Weiss and Baker, 1933). In addition, baroreceptor stimulation also produces cortical and behavioral inhibition (Bonvallet et al, 1953; Lacey et al, 1963; Lacey and Lacey, 1974). For example, Dworkin et al (1979) raised blood pressure in rats by infusion of phenylephrine; they found that rats showed less running to terminate or avoid noxious stimuli than during saline infusions.

Hernandez-Peon (1964) and Silverman (1967) were the first to suggest how such increases in blood pressure might serve to effect an ideal form of psychological defensiveness. That is, sensory thresholds were lowered, leading to an increased awareness of the sensory aspects of stimulus events and configurations. Since the brain has limited capacity to process information, enhanced processing of sensory information implies depressed processing of cognitive-ideational information, hence effecting defense against psychologically disturbing cognitions.

The suggestion is that some instances of high blood pressure in adults might be considered a secondary homeostatic compensatory response by an excessively automatized (bored) brain to de-automatize itself; that is, the bored brain may increase its awareness of the *sensory* information in the environment by increasing the blood pressure. The implication is that some forms of hypertension can be treated by providing the hypertensive individual interesting environments and/or activities, as well as by teaching of techniques (meditational) which effect de-automatization of attentional processes. The psychophysiological approach suggests that the current medical emphasis on medication in the treatment of hypertension is in need of closer scrutiny in regards to the validity of its rationale and its outlook (e.g. that *all* hypertension must be controlled and brought down by medication to some normal range).

Cancer

Evidence reviewed in Chapter 3 pointed out the association between low levels of CNS information flow and carcinogenesis in epithelial tissue. Carcinogenesis, in turn, was construed to represent the genesis of novelty or information which initially increases information flow as cells metastasize and take over functions in other bodily parts. Later, in the terminal stages, the severe pain resulting from tumors pressing on surrounding nerves is also fed-back to the brain, effecting increases in sensory information flow for the cortex, but having a maladaptive effect for the integrity of the whole body.

Miscellaneous Somatic Disorders

My hypothesis suggests that many other somatic disorders may, in some instances, be conceptualized as homeostatic, "fail-safe" processes which help to rectify significant mismatch of optimal information load for the cortex. For example, allergies, hernia, some types of hyperthyroidism, etc., are posited to be associated with increments in cognitive structure and to be exacerbated when the cortex is experiencing considerable information underload. All of these disorders increase the amount of endogenous information processing for the brain, e.g., the itching, inflammation of allergies; the pain of hernia; and the general, sympathetic nervous system activation of hyperthyroidism.

Behavioral Phenomena

Violence, Explosive and Hyperactive Behavior

Aggression and violence continue to be one of the major public health problems. In 1968, more Americans were the victims of murder and aggravated assault in the United States than were killed and wounded in seven-and-one-half years of the Vietnam war; almost half a million Americans were the victims of homicide, rape, and assault. Many people today are afraid to venture out on city streets at night for fear of personal attack; new violence victims continue to be treated daily at major emergency or receiving hospitals in every city of the United States (Mark and Ervin, 1970). Apparently, much of the violence is done for thrills and out of a sense of boredom and futility (cf. de la Peña, 1979). One way of rectifying the low intensity of consciousness, which is a consequence of increments in phylogenetic and ontogenetic experience, is to engage the environment in a more vigorous fashion, hence to augment sensory information flow to the understimulated brain (de la Peña, 1971; 1978; 1979).

Some neurological and psychophysiological studies suggest that the gross, impulsive, and often, aggressive motor behavior displayed in certain behavioral disorders such as the hyperkinetic syndrome of childhood (Satterfield and Dawson, 1971; Satterfield et al, 1972; Spring et al, 1974) and adulthood psychopathy (Quay, 1966; Hare, 1975; Mednick, 1975; Borkovec, 1970) may represent an extreme form of stimulus-seeking behavior which attempts to compensate for low levels of physiological activation and/or sensory stimulation obtaining for a relatively insensitive, waking perceptual apparatus. It has been proposed, for example, that the low level of spontaneous electrodermal activity found among psychopaths in several studies is indicative of chronic autonomic and cortical hypoarousal and that this might account for both stimulus seeking tendencies (Hare, 1975) and role-taking deficiencies (Schalling, 1978).

The point of view taken here and elsewhere (de la Peña, 1979a) is that much of the hyperactive, explosive behavior observed in our sophisticated Western society is an attempt by the excessively auto-matized brain to rectify the aberrantly low level of information flow which obtains with increments in experience. That is, owing to the greater efficiency of our evolved brains in processing information, less surprisal or information obtains in transactions with ordinary environ-ments. The sequela is a low intensity of consciousness which can be rectified, to some extent, by engaging in frenetic and/or violent activity since the result is an augmentation of the overall information processing rate.

Wilson (1979: 525) has captured the argument expressed here:

> In short, man's success in achieving "self-auto-mation" has now become the chief obstacle to his evolution. Gurdjieff once said that if the human race is to be saved, man must develop an organ that would enable him to foresee the precise hour and moment of his own death. That would stir him out of his laziness. Auden was pointing to the same

defect when he said: "Even war cannot frighten us
enough."

Alcoholism and Stimulant Drug Abuse

Stimulant drug abuse (nicotine, caffeine, amphetamines, alcohol, marijuana, cocaine, etc.) is conceptualized to occur in response to excessive automatization of attentional processes. Studies of the effects of
alcohol and various stimulant drugs on indices of central and autonomic nervous system activation indicate that these drugs *initially*
induce CNS activating effects. On the other hand, they frequently are
reported to *reduce* behavioral and self-report measures of anxiety and
to effect feelings of increased tranquility (cf. Gilbert, 1979). This
general pattern of increased physiological activation coupled with
decreased phenomenological activation (anxiety) has been extensively
documented for all of the aforementioned stimulant drugs, perhaps
most extensively for nicotine (Frith, 1971; Ikard, Green and Horn,
1969; Ikard and Thompkins, 1973).

This apparent paradox of increasing physiological activation being
associated with decreases in self-reports of anxiety is hypothesized to
obtain thus: excessive automatization of attentional processes results
in a condition of functional sensory information deprivation. When
information flow becomes excessively low, i.e., boredom and anxiety is
experienced, the brain seeks out activities or chemicals which rectify
the aberrantly low levels of physiological activation and phenomenological anxiety. In our highly evolved society, stimulant drugs such as
alcohol (initially a stimulant, later a depressant), marijuana, nicotine,
cocaine, caffeine, are easily obtained; they quickly but temporarily
rectify aberrantly low levels of physiological activation and hence
reduce the experience of "anxiety," since positive affect (relaxation,
interest) is apparently associated with some intermediate range/rate
of information flow.

However, after the effects of the drug terminate, the CNS
returns to a level below its already aberrantly low baseline, because
the nervous system seems to act like a rubber band; *stretches*
(ergotropic activation) are generally followed by compensatory *relaxation* (trophotropic activation). The result is a vicious cycle of
caffeine, nicotine, marijuana intake followed by a let-down, which
initiates further drug ingestion, and then the problem of addiction
arises. Moreover, with chronic use, various non-CNS organs begin to
suffer damage (sometimes irreparable), e.g., nicotine and marijuana
damage the lungs; alcohol, the liver. Thus, while the brain and CNS
continue to receive adaptive increments in information flow for
organized function from the effects of the drugs, various non-CNS
structures begin to suffer damage and debilitation, often leading to
death of the organism (e.g., lung cancer, cirrhosis of the liver,
bleeding ulcers, cardiovascular disease).

Some Varieties of Schizophrenia

Literature review in Chapter 3 indicates that the performance of heterogeneous groups of schizophrenics tends to define the extremes on several basic response dimensions, including sensitivity to sensory stimulation (de la Peña, 1971; Fischer et al, 1968; Silverman, 1968) and levels of physiological activation (Claridge and Hume, 1966; Depue and Fowles, 1974; Lang and Buss, 1965; Venables, 1964). The disordered perceptual, cognitive, and behavioral function of schizophrenia can thus be associated with the information underload and/or information overload experienced by the majority of such patients. That is, the good, premorbid, behaviorally-hyperactive, paranoid schizophrenic is posited to experience significant information underload in the pre-morbid state. The hyperactive behavior, hallucinations and delusions all serve to rectify aberrantly low levels of information flow, often a consequence of too low a level of environmental information flow for a relatively high level of development of cortical structure. The opposite set of conditions is posited to be the case for the poor premorbid, behaviorally-hypoactive non-paranoid schizophrenic.

Some Types of Depression and Suicide

It is posited that automatization of attentional processes is at the core of depression and suicide (including chronic unsuccessful suicide attempts). There is much evidence that many forms of depression may be associated with abnormally low levels of sensory flow and activation. During the 1950s, a number of reports indicated that depression often developed in patients being treated with reserpine, a drug which markedly lowers sensory flow and activation. Drugs that cause depletion and inactivation of norepinephrine (NE) in the CNS often produce depression, while drugs which increase NE are associated with an anti-depressant effect (Schildkraut and Kety, 1967). Generally NE enhances physiological activation, as measured by various peripheral and central indices in men and animals. In addition, there is experimental work showing that under hypnosis, if anger on one occasion and relaxation and depression on another are suggested, the subject shows an adrenergic (sympathetic autonomic nervous system dominance mediated by NE) reaction to anger and a cholinergic (dominance of parasympathetic autonomic nervous system mediated by acetylcholine) response to depression and relaxation as shown by respiratory and metabolic indicators (Dudley et al, 1964). Electroconvulsive therapy (ECT), which has strong activating effects, often is used successfully in the treatment of some forms of depression, implying that certain depressives may be in a state of abnormally low physiological activation which is rectified by the excitatory effects of ECT (Gellhorn and Kiely, 1973). Waking psychophysiological studies by Dawson et al (1977) and others (Lader and Wing, 1969; Noble and Lader, 1971; Kelly and Walter, 1968; Lader and Noble, 1975) point out that low autonomic activation, as indexed by low levels of basal skin conductance and number of spontaneous skin resistance changes, is characteristic of the depressed state (there is conflicting data for other physiological measures, however).

Post-Traumatic (Vietnam) Delayed Stress Syndrome

This syndrome is characterized by a host of mental, physical and behavioral difficulties following participation in the Vietnam conflict. A salient aspect of the syndrome is its delay in appearance. Apparently most of these individuals were able to maintain a high degree of psychophysiological integrity *during* their service, when life-threatening occurrences were a part of day-to-day existence. Rather, the problems generally emerge *after* the danger and unpredictable circumstances have ended and the demands upon the individual for survival-optimizing activity have been relieved.

I posit that a large part of this phenomenon may be conceptualized along information underload lines. That is, the individual who has the greatest chance of developing the syndrome is one who has a relatively high need for stimulating, information-rich environments. When this individual is removed from the relatively unpredictable informative wartime environment, he experiences a phenomenon not unlike sensory deprivation and/or boredom. The consequence is that the understimulated brain then modulates information flow to higher levels by promotion of behavioral, psychological, and somatic processes which increase the sensory information flow (pain syndromes, sleep disturbances, psychosis, neurosis, excessive cognitive rumination, etc.). What differentiates the syndrome from the World War I, World War II, and Korean experience is probably the relative interpersonal isolation that most Vietnam veterans must endure upon their return home. That is, while returning veterans from other wars were given much attention (stimulation) and adulation upon their return, returning Vietnam veterans were largely ignored. The lack of interpersonal stimulation, coupled with a lower socio-economic level which largely precludes engaging in interesting work or vocations, further compounds the problem of information underload.

Change for the Sake of Change

It is posited that many phenomena which are endemic to Western society—serial monogamy, frequent changes in jobs, incessant purchasing of new products and items, the great need for travel—in large part reflect our rapid habituation to our environments. That is, automatization and boredom escalate as we gain experience with the environment; as a consequence, we engage in attempts to rectify automatization of attention by discarding the old and acquiring the new, whether mates or material objects. This often has disastrous consequences for the maintenance of self, bank accounts, and society (witness inflation, credit card mania, and the general paranoia and sense of emptiness that pervades a large part of contemporary society).

Overpopulation

Although it is difficult to decide how intense the desire and ability to procreate offspring must be before it becomes maladaptive for self and society, there is no doubt that some individuals seem disposed to create large numbers of progeny. Obviously while cultural or religious beliefs can play a role in such behavior, it is posited that often such behavior may reflect excessive automatization of attentional processes, i.e., boredom, loneliness, depression, etc., which can be rectified to some extent by the creation of novelty (new individuals). The young child may be viewed as providing de-automatization for the excessively automatized adult. De-automatization is provided by crises precipitated by the child's helplessness and vulnerability, and from the adult's vicariously re-discovering, through the child's relatively de-automatized perceptions, parts of the world to which adults have become habituated and which they have learned to ignore (e.g., sensory impressions, playful, illogical thoughts and perceptions).

Varieties of Religious Practices

Various forms of religious practice may be viewed in terms of automatization-deautomatization (Wilson, 1957). The Gurdjieff School (Wilson, 1978) emphasizes the practice of activities which appear to have a de-automatizing function. That is, when Gurdjieff's religious ascetics wore hair shirts and slept on bare planks, or were awakened from sleep and expected to perform complex motor activities immediately, it was because Gurdjieff recognized instinctively that the central problem is deconditioning from over reliance on activities and cognition made habitual by repeated practice. In essence, the ascetics were trying to shake the robotic mind awake through pain and discomfort.

Some of the practices and teachings of Jesus and modern day Christianity may also be viewed within an attentional framework (Wilson, 1957). For example, the practice of giving thanks and/or verbalizing appreciation of ordinary objects in the environment (e.g., "grace" before meals, giving thanks for one's health and family, etc., before sleep) may be considered modes of investing attention or consciousness in activities and/or objects generally rendered unconscious by repeated experience. Similarly, the practice of giving care and attention to the ill and less fortunate may be considered attentional devices for self-remembering and/or investing interest in the environment, i.e., bringing to consciousness the fact that one is fortunate in having relatively better health or circumstance than the one cared for (Willingham, 1981).

Other aspects of religious activities may also be conceptualized within an attentional framework. It seems likely that the mantras, chants, and other stereotyped activity (dance, prayer) employed by various religious groups may serve the function of narrowing attention in order to capitalize on the compensatory broadening of attention which obtains following these activities (Naranjo and Ornstein, 1971).

HEALTH PHENOMENA ASSOCIATED WITH LOW LEVELS OF EXPERIENCE

Somatic Phenomena

Some Forms of Hypertension

There are undoubtedly some forms of hypertension in which the elevated blood pressure does not involve a brain control process to help rectify sensory information underload.   Rather heterostasis is implied. For example, an organism with an imbalance in the direction of sympathetic dominance (and/or lack of inhibitory neural circuitry) would constantly be orienting to environmental sensory stimuli. The result would be sustained increases in blood pressure which eventually would become permanent.   Many subgroups of mentally retarded individuals show hypertension as a cardinal feature (e.g., Turner's syndrome, mongoloids, frontally brain damaged individuals). Excessive de-automatization, associated with failure to form mental models of stimulus configurations and/or contingencies, would be more likely found in the less experienced or evolved organism; these individuals would likely be behaviorally hypoactive, show low sensory thresholds, and be autonomically hyperaroused relative to organisms having more development of cognitive (cortical) structure.

Some Varieties of Cancer

As outlined in Chapter 3, some varieties of cancer (certain types of leukemia, some types of carcinomas and sarcomas) seem to develop in response to severe information overload; that is, when the brain experiences severe information overload it "switches in" a compensatory state of information underload to protect itself from the information inundation. The information underload state is the necessary condition for the genesis of "new" information which is the cancer cell.

Certain Psychophysiological Disorders in Children

Children have relatively low levels of development of cognitive structure relative to mature adults. According to premises of the mismatch hypothesis, children should thus be more susceptible than adults to "information-overload" induced illnesses. Unfortunately, the entire area of psychosomatic problems in children is vague and in need of much more research (Finch, 1977). However, it is quite clear that certain infectious diseases (colds, chicken pox, mumps, etc.), and certain types of cancer (see Chapter 2) appear much more frequently in children relative to older individuals. It is hypothesized that these illnesses occur following periods of time when there is too much information and/or stimulation for the child's relatively underdeveloped cortex and/or immunological system. The result is a relatively rapid exhaustion of anti-inflammatory hormonal capacity (there is little redundancy relative to older organisms) and the switching-in of compensatory homeostatic pro-inflammatory hormonal processes to eliminate viruses, bacteria, etc., which have enjoyed easy entry into bodily tissues.

Behavioral Phenomena

There are sundry behavioral phenomena ostensibly associated with low levels of development of cognitive structure and/or excessive deautomatization.

Some Varieties of Mental Retardation

Defects in amino acid metabolism are often associated with mental retardation. Phenylketonuria (PKU) is one of the best defined of the amino acid defects. An estimated 98% of PKU patients, if untreated, will show IQ's of less than 60 (Stanbury et al, 1966). Approximately 60% of the patients have microcephaly, hyperactive monosynaptic reflexes and an inability to talk. While psychophysiological studies of PKU and other aminoacidopathies associated with mental retardation are lacking, the fact that most can be treated by low protein diets or by withholding certain amino acids from the diet (Barness et al, 1973) implies a disorder involving excessively high physiological activation. This is because diets rich in protein have been found to increase circulating levels of the excitatory CNS neurotransmitter norepinephrine in the brain (Fernstrom and Wurtman, 1972; 1974).

Some Types of Schizophrenia

Literature review in Chapter 3 pointed out the existence of two very different types of schizophrenics. As previously noted earlier in this chapter, literature review suggests that the good pre-morbid, hyperactive paranoid schizophrenic has the problem of information underload owing to a relatively high level of development of cognitive structure. In contrast, there is evidence that the poor pre-morbid behaviorally hypoactive non-paranoid schizophrenic has the problem of information overload owing to a relatively low level of development of cognitive structure. That is, the latter may be characterized to be hypersensitive to incoming sensory stimulation since he has little cognitive structure through which he may filter the environment. Catatonia and behavioral hypoactivity represent the brain's attempt to rectify information overload by minimizing the information processing which normally accompanies behavior.

In support of this model of schizophrenia, Mirsky (1969) studied the brains of post-mortem schizophrenics. Mirsky (1969) presents a neuropsychological theory of schizophrenia which is consonant with the view offered here. In reviewing the many studies, he tries to make a case for two basically distinct types of brain pathology in schizophrenia. In the poor pre-morbid, non-paranoid cases, he suggests that the brain pathology is one of long standing that may be associated in part with diffuse *frontal* lobe damage including destruction of tissue in ventral and orbital areas and associated subcortical structures such as the medialis dorsalis of the thalamus and the head of the caudate nucleus (Blum et al, 1950). In the good pre-morbid or episodic paranoid group, on the other hand, the damage may preferentially be found in septal, hippocampal and temporal lobe (*posterior* cortex) areas (Heath, 1964a; 1964b).

Some Forms of Drug Abuse

Finally, it is posited that some forms of alcoholism and some types of CNS depressant drug abuse are associated with low levels of development of cognitive structure and/or excessive deautomatization of attentional processes. Alcohol, for example, has an ascending (CNS stimulating) as well as a descending (CNS depressing) "arm" (Jones et al, 1976). It seems likely that excessively deautomatized individuals drink alcohol primarily for its CNS depressing effect. Such individuals might likely become dependent on other CNS depressant drugs such as the minor and major tranquilizers, heroin, and morphine. In these cases, the overexcited, overloaded brain learns quickly that these drugs effect a decrease in anxiety and promote perceptual-cognitive-behavioral organization. The problem is that, with continued use, tolerance develops and larger doses are required to produce the same relaxing effect. Drug dependence then develops and becomes problematic.

Some Types of Violent, Aggressive Behavior and Hypersexuality

Some forms of explosive, violent, aggressive behavior are probably associated with information overload and/or excessive deautomatization. In these cases, controls, i.e., the "turning down" of behavior in order to rectify information overload, are inoperative. The result is a massive discharge of behavior since excessive behavior and the accompanying increments in information processing will eventually be followed by a compensatory decrease in information processing, exhaustion and/or death.

Neurological studies lend support to this point of view. Disease or damage to the frontal lobes in humans frequently is associated with hypersexuality (Hafner, 1957; Jarvie, 1954; Lauber, 1958), hyperorality, and hyperphagia (Fulton et al, 1932; Watts and Fulton, 1934; Langworthy and Richter, 1939). It seems reasonable to view these behaviors as occurring in excess amounts and intensities because the increments in information flow in one "arm" of each type of behavior (e.g., pre-orgasmic phase of sexual behavior, orality and the ingestion of food, intense behavior), is followed by decrements in information flow in the second phase (e.g., post-orgasmic phase of sexual behavior, the somnolence following meals, the exhaustion after periods of intense behavioral activity).

SUMMARY

This chapter reviewed evidence which suggests a possible homeostatic function for many of the psychological, somatic, and behavioral disorders which afflict contemporary man. That is, there is much evidence to support the view that the overly automatized brain may employ illness behavior and sequelæ as mechanisms for enhancing information flow when information flow is at sub-optimal levels. Literature review also points out that some forms of these disorders are heterostatic for organized brain function and are probably reflective of a more pervasive organismic heterostasis.

While infectious disease was not considered in my review, it seems likely that some instances of infectious disorder are modulated by mismatch at the cortical level. For example, it is a common observation that colds and flu often follow disappointing, depressing, and boring experiences, as well as the converse condition of overwhelming excitement and happiness. In the former case the bored brain apparently modulates an enhanced information flow rate for itself by promoting the viability of an infectious process. The common cold, for example, provides a certain amount of information to the brain by increasing the brain's awareness of somatic structures which are normally out of awareness. Most of us are generally unaware of information flow in the nose, throat, chest and head until an infectious process makes its presence felt there.

Other varieties of infectious processes may reflect a generalized state of organismic deautomatization. That is, the augmented information flow for the cortex relative to the pre-infectious state may reflect the generalized failure of homeostatic mechanisms in an organism headed for a hasty demise. On the other hand, conceivably there are some varieties of infectious disorder which are homeostatic for the excessively de-automatized brain, in that the cortical information flow rate provided by the relatively isolated environment is substantially lower relative to the pre-morbid environment.

Finally, it is probable that mismatch theory is applicable at the level of immunological structure. For example, an exotic stimulus such as BCG will provide a high degree of information flow for immunological structures which do not have prior experience with BCG. On the other hand, there is the suggestion that highly developed immunological structures in contact with ordinary antigenic environments may experience something akin to information underload; the presence of allergic reactions may connote a form of paranoia at the cellular level which acts to redress cortical information underload.

Chapter 9 Extensions of Mismatch Theory to Sleep and Sexual Disorders and the Phenomenon of Death

Under atypical circumstances, dreams may be repetitive or use stereotyped visual idioms, but the general rule is that we surprise ourselves with what we dream. Each dream contains images which we literally did not conceive that we could conceive.

David Foulkes
A Grammar of Dreams

★ ★ ★

I'm growing old! I'm falling apart! And it's VERY INTEREST-ING!

William Saroyan

INTRODUCTION

The last chapter described application of mismatch theory to a broad range of somatic and behavioral phenomena. It points out the possibility that many health-related phenomena, traditionally viewed by the medical establishment as disorder, may, in certain instances, play a homeostatic adaptive role in effecting optimal levels/rates of informational processing for the excessively automatized brain, albeit often at the expense of the integrity (ordered function) of sub- or supra-structures within the hierarchy of organizational structures comprising the organism.

This chapter extends the argument to a broad range of sleep and sexual disorders. Evidence is reviewed which suggests that some varieties of sleep and sexual disorders may be conceptualized as homeostatic compensatory behaviors and/or processes by which the excessively automatized (bored) brain rectifies suboptimal levels of waking sensory information flow to higher, more optimal levels for organized waking perceptual-cognitive-behavioral function and the experience of relaxation/positive affect.

INSOMNIA

Insomnia usually refers to complaints of poor sleep, unrefreshing sleep, abbreviated sleep, sleep punctuated by abnormal restlessness, and interrupted sleep. Research findings on insomnia are inconsistent and have been reviewed in detail elsewhere (de la Peña, 1978). It is suggested that mismatch theory can bring order to a wealth of contradictory and inconsistent findings.

Mismatch theory suggests that when the rate of overall information processing in the CNS is within the optimal range needed for organized waking perceptual-cognitive-behavioral function, there is a direct positive correlation between rate of overall information processing in the CNS and propensity for the behavioral state of wakefulness. That is, when overall information processing is within the optimal range needed for organized function, a relatively low information processing rate is conducive to sleep onset and maintenance. (Figure 3)

Difficulty in sleep initiation and maintenance (insomnia) is hypothesized to obtain when the overall rate of information processing in the CNS is high. Insomnia is the sleep behavior sequela of *severe* information underload (chronic, severe boredom) *or* information overload (excitement), the former condition "switching in" a compensatory high rate of information flow for cortical homeostasis which is too high for sleep to obtain. (Figure 3)

It is suggested that many apparent paradoxical or discrepant findings on sleep-waking sensory flow and activation interrelations are resolved by the proffered approach. The model can explain the paradoxical sleep behaviors that often obtain with extreme levels of information underload or overload. For example, changes in proclivity for sleep with varying durations of waking sensory deprivation become more understandable. That is, the general finding is that sleep is often excessive early in the sensory deprivation period (Potter and Heron, 1972; Royal, 1976), i.e., the first day or two. As the deprivation continues, however, sleep either returns to normal values with respect to total sleep-time and sleep stage distribution but with increased phasic REM density (Potter and Heron, 1972, four to seven days of deprivation), or there is a reduction in mean total sleep-time per twenty-four hours (Royal, 1976, mean of last two of seven-day deprivation). These findings and other similar reports (Ware, 1976) suggest that low-level waking sensory flow and activation is initially conducive to sleep onset and maintenance. If the amount of sensory flow and activation falls outside some optimal range over some relatively protracted temporal interval, e.g., is *excessively* low, the brain takes steps to rectify the low level sensory flow and activation by increasing the sensory flow and activation obtaining during REM sleep periods and/or by increasing the information flow rate to a high enough level to preclude sleep onset and/or maintenance. (Figure 3)

Paradoxical observations (Oswald, 1960; Oswald, 1962) that extremely high-level, waking sensory flow and activation often effect

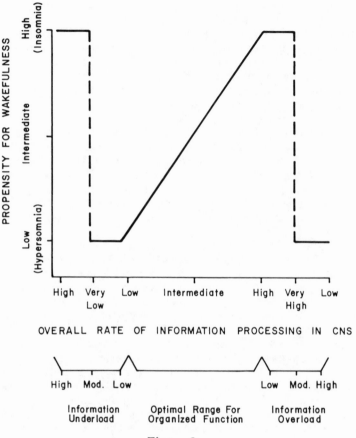

Figure 3

efficient sleep onset and maintenance may be explained within the framework. When the waking brain experiences extremely high level sensory flow and activation, it switches in a compensatory, homeostatic, sensory, information-*reducing* state of consciousness via the utilization of various brain waking sensory control processes, e.g., elevated sensory thresholds, behavioral hypoactivity, low activation in various physiological subsystems, etc.   The result is that waking sensory flow and activation drops to low levels which are commensurate with sleep and the individual may experience hypersomnia or a high propensity for sleep. On the other hand, chronically understimulating environments are often observed to produce a paradoxical alerting effect accompanied by anxiety.   Weybrew (1961) observed insomnia and anxiety in men who were living in the information-poor Antarctic environment. Apparently the understimulated brain rectifies the information underload by initiating physiological and behavioral processes which provide too high a level of information flow for sleep onset and maintenance.

The hypothesis suggests that studies reporting no effects (Bonnett and Webb, 1976; Frederickson et al, 1969; Hauri, 1969; Webb and Friedman, 1971) of variations in waking sensory flow on sleep may have effected extreme rates of information processing in the CNS, so that the brain employed *waking*, sensory modulating mechanisms exclusively and expediently to keep sensory flow within the optimal range needed for organized waking perceptual-cognitive-behavioral function; or compensatory sleep sensory regulating responses to waking sensory manipulations may have occurred in variables other than those chosen for study (e.g. phasic REM intensity, density).

Disparate findings vis-à-vis first night effects might be explained in part by individual differences in sensory regulating characteristics. I found that insomniac individuals showing reverse first night effects showed higher sensation-seeking scores, more self-rated boredom, and smoked more cigarettes per day compared to normal first-night effect insomniacs (de la Peña, 1977). These findings, recently replicated by Hauri and Olmstead (1981), imply that some chronic insomniacs may be in a state of chronic sensory information underload (boredom) which is anxiety producing. The enhanced sensory flow and activation obtaining in response to the novel, first-night sleep lab environment raises the aberrantly low ˙sensory flow and activation to some level that is within the optimal range needed for organized cortical function and for feelings of relaxation. Thus, chronically bored insomniacs sleep better the first night in the lab; on subsequent nights, boredom, and subsequently, anxiety, mitigates against sleep.

In situational (environmental) insomnia, normally efficient sleepers experience temporary stresses which sometimes effect levels of waking sensory flow exceeding or falling short of the optimal range needed for efficient sleep. Some of these temporary episodes are associated with too high a level of sensory flow, e.g., Christmas Eve for many children, an athlete on the eve of an important tournament, wives of returning veterans losing sleep out of anticipation, one's moving to a new city. Other temporary episodes may provide too low a level of sensory flow for efficient sleep to obtain, e.g., the death or loss of a beloved person, wherein the loss is one of stimulation and/or information as well, losing a job and having nothing to do during the day, experiencing a dearth of daytime physical activity subsequent to breaking a leg. In chronic (constitutional) insomnia, the individual manifests relatively chronic abnormal and/or disorganized sleep parameters-patterns associated with relatively chronic information overload and/or information underload in waking sensory information processing systems.

Neurotic insomnia is characterized by obsessive worrying and thinking. Many self-defined insomniacs report remembering a great many thoughts running through their minds prior to sleep as well as during early non-REM sleep (Rechtschaffen and Monroe, 1969). One consequence is feeling awake even though asleep according to EEG criteria. Active, obsessive worrying may be associated with more information flow than the more passive hypnagogic fantasy that usually precedes sleep (Coursey, 1975). The developmental psycho-physiological approach and mismatch theory suggest that excessive cognitive-ideational rumination is often a compensatory brain response to sensory information underload. The finding that monotonous tones, background music, and white noise helps many neurotic insomniacs sleep is consistent with the mismatch theory of insomnia because the enhanced sensory flow and activation provided by moderate-level external stimulation increases the aberrantly low sensory flow and activation to within the optimal range needed for organized sleep-wakefulness function, and thus diminishes the need for excessive cognitive-ideational stimulation.

The insomnia of old age is readily conceptualizeable within the described theoretical framework. Evidence reviewed previously sug-gested that old age is associated with decreased sensory flow and activation in most somatic systems. Old age is associated with decrements in physical and motor capacities. However, studies of cognitive function in gerontological populations (Owens, 1959; Schaie and Strother, 1964) suggest that decrements in cognitive abilities are not as large as decrements obtaining in sensory processing capacities. The suggestion is that in old age the CNS experiences a high degree of functional sensory information underload, since CNS structure is relatively intact (a relatively high degree of cognitive ability is apparently maintained) and thus still needs a relatively high level of information processing for organized perceptual-cognitive-behavioral function. However, the usual channels for supplying a large portion of the information (e.g., sensory information channels, including behav-ioral activity-related sensory information channels) are capable of providing only a limited amount of the optimal range needed for organized brain function. The resulting sensory information underload is associated with the insomnia of old age and is manifested polygraph-ically as an exaggeration of changes in sleep architecture normally obtaining with increments in psychological depression. At least one index of physiological activation increases with age, blood pressure. Thus, old age is associated with extremes of sensory flow and activation in the various systems of the body; in some cases, incre-ments in blood pressure may serve to increase the brain's sensory gain and hence rectify the sensory underload associated with aging.

Insomnia is often associated with nocturnal myoclonus, a condition characterized by the occurrence during sleep of periodic episodes of repititive and stereotyped leg muscle jerks. Insomnia is also often associated with restless legs syndrome since the afflicted individual feels extremely disagreeable, creeping sensations inside the calves whenever sitting or lying down. The dysesthesias are rarely painful, but agonizingly unremitting, and cause an almost irresistible urge to move the legs, thus interefering with sleep. Apparently the relatively high level of sensory flow and activation accompanying these motor automatisms (Lugaresi et al, 1967) is sufficient to disturb sleep continuity, i.e., partial or full arousals or awakenings often obtain. The possibility of homeostatic and heterostatic varieties of each syndrome exists; that is, boredom during wakefulness may be rectified by the increased information flow effected by nocturnal myoclonus (homeostatic). In *heterostatic* myoclonus, the enhanced information flow associated with the abnormal motor activity during sleep would be reflective of the generalized decrement in inhibitory cortical processes which accompanies increasing systemic entropy (as in old age).

Sleep psychophysiology in depression is consistent with the hypothesis of excessive automatization. The most consistent characteristics of sleep in depressed patients are: absence or marked decrease of stage 4 sleep (Hauri, 1974; Hawkins and Mendels, 1966); short latencies to the first REM period (Coble et al, 1976; Kupfer and Foster, 1972); abnormal distributions of REMs within a REM period (Hauri & Hawkins, 1971; Snyder, 1972); large intraindividual variability in phasic REM intensity across nights (Snyder, 1972); a tendency for higher REM densities in primary compared to secondary depression (Foster et al, 1967); fragmentation of sleep characterized by frequent awakenings and disordered sleep cycles (Hawkins et al, 1967; Zung et al, 1964); and early morning awakenings.

If most forms of depression can be assumed to be associated with abnormally low levels of sensory flow and activation, and if information underload is associated with aberrant or disorganized sleep function, the relation of insomnia with depression is clarified. For example, low amounts of stage 4 sleep obtain because the "primary" depressed individual is experiencing low level sensory flow and activation during wakefulness, i.e., there is a little need (in the homeostatic sense) for the low level sensory flow and activation accompanying slow wave sleep. Latencies to the first REM sleep period are short because the sleeping brain attempts to rectify the low level waking sensory flow and activation as quickly as possible. Intraindividual variations in phasic REM densities from night to night might be associated with homeostatic CNS influences in the depressive episode. Phasic REM intensities-densities would be higher in primary as opposed to secondary depression, because the latter condition is associated with considerably more waking sensory flow and activation associated with the pain of medical problems and surgical procedures, stresses of life-threatening medical conditions, stimulation provided by toxic and infectious states, etc. Frequent awakenings conceivably would occur to increase the probability of sensory flow and activation since wakefulness generally provides comparable sensory flow and activation to REM sleep (Johnson, 1973) and certainly more than that obtaining during NREM sleep. Early morning awakenings (occurring frequently after the second or third REM period of the night) occur because (a) the brain seeks to maintain the relatively high sensory flow and activation it has just achieved and/or (b) the REM sleep periods may have reached some limit with respect to the amount of endogenous sensory flow and activation they can provide during sleep, i.e., it is possible that after four to five hours of sleep the brain of the depressed individual has reached some upper limit of endogenous sensory flow and activation that can occur during sleep (which normals experience after seven to eight hours of sleep). This upper limit is indexed by some maximum value of phasic REM density and/or intensity, signaling "sleep satiety" (Aserinsky, 1969) to the brain, and wakefulness obtains. In addition, total sleep deprivation (cf. Larsen et al, 1976) or REM sleep deprivation (cf. Vogel et al, 1975) would effect therapeutic results since both procedures increase the overall twenty-four-hour sensory flow and activation to that obtaining in the normal sleep-wakefulness cycle (e.g., both total sleep and REM deprivation effect considerable reduction of NREM "sensory-informa-tion-reducing" sleep and provide much stimulation-stress during the enforced awakenings).

Finally, improvements in sleep in many depressed individuals following the administration of "activating" anti-depressant drugs and stimulant medications is consistent with the mismatch theory: the abnormally low level of sensory flow and activation associated with excessive automatization of waking attentional processes is rectified by the increased sensory flow obtaining with the administration of CNS-stimulating drugs so that information flow falls within the optimal range needed for organized sleep-waking function and for the experience of relaxation.

The observation that the withdrawal of alcohol, hypnotic and psychotropic drugs is often associated with heightened sensory flow, physiological activation and insomnia is consistent with the mismatch theory of insomnia. For example, sensory information overload manifested as hallucinations often accompanies alcohol withdrawal and is associated with extreme anxiety and heightened physiological activation, including extremely high sensory flow and activation occurring during REM sleep periods. Thus, too high a level of sensory flow and activation obtains for the efficient onset and maintenance of sleep.

EXCESSIVE SLEEPINESS AND HYPERSOMNIA

Narcolepsy and sleep apnea are the most common disorders character-ized by an excessive propensity for sleep. Mismatch theory suggests that excessive automatization of attention is at the root of the problem. Sleep patterns in classical narcolepsy overlap greatly with those found in depressive syndromes (e.g., diminished deep sleep, short latencies to REM sleep, fragmentation of sleep); the same is true for waking psychophysiological patterns (e.g., constricted pupils, low skin conductance levels). Narcolepsy is late to develop in ontogeny and phylogeny and thus is associated with high degrees of automatization of perceptual and physiological processes, the result being a "low intensity of consciousness, boredom, sleepiness, fatigue, etc." In keeping with this hypothesis, narcoleptics generally score higher than population norms on intelligence tests and are generally over-repre-sented in scientific and technical fields (de la Peña, 1980a). Narcolepsy may be associated with constitutionally determined, low sensory information flow levels and low levels of CNS activation due to dominance of cholinergic processes (Gellhorn and Kiely 1973; de la Peña, 1977). Anecdotal reports from narcoleptics indicate that the experience of depression exacerbates the symptomology. The cardinal sleep features of narcolepsy apparently act to rectify the low amount and/or rate of waking sensory information flow experienced by the waking brain. That is, the narcoleptic quickly enters sensory information-rich REM sleep periods, and experiences many awakenings which provide increments in amounts of sensory information flow. Sensory information-poor NREM sleep is generally by-passed. Cataplexy (loss of muscle tone) represents a rebound of excessive trophotropic (parasympathetic) activity following ergotropic (sympathetic) activity (anger, laughter, surprise) in a trophotropically-tuned nervous system.

Sleep apnea is a condition in which the individual suffers respiratory impairment during sleep. In obstructive apnea, there is a collapse or blockage of the airway at the level of the pharynx so that, although respiratory effort is made, there is no exchange of air. Most of these individuals are males and obese. Their most common complaint is excessive daytime sleepiness, although a few complain chiefly about poor sleep (associated with arousals following blockage of airflow).

My colleague J. Fisher (Fisher, 1977) has found, in many cases, that weight gain in these individuals followed a life event which was perceived by the patients as stressful and depressing. I suggest that the excessive weight gain is due to excessive dominance of trophotropic (anabolic) processes mediated by depressing environmental events in trophotropically-tuned individuals; the result is the building up of excessive fatty tissue in the throat which blocks the airflow when the patient relaxes sufficiently (as during sleep). Another possible mechanism is the excessive relaxation (hypotonus) of the muscles in the oropharanx associated with excessively low physiological activation in trophotropically-tuned individuals during sleep.

The awakenings/arousals which occur following apnea periods during sleep (Guilleminault et al, 1973) are conceptualized to effect increments in sensory information flow and/or physiological activation and are considered to help compensate for the excessively low levels of sensory information flow during wakefulness associated with excessive automatization of attentional processes (boredom). This notion would help explain recent findings (McGinty et al, 1981) that a rocking bed, which provides increments in sensory information flow relative to a stationary bed, facilitates diaphragmatic EMG activity during both NREM and REM sleep in sleeping kittens. That is, vestibular stimulation apparently modulates endogenous sensory information flow to higher levels and facilitates respiration during sleep. Such findings, if replicable with humans, suggest that increments in sensory information flow during sleep may decrease the need for information flow concomitant with apnea periods, and may be of therapeutic value in the amelioration of central sleep apnea.

Moreover, since the apneas effect partial sleep deprivation, particularly of deep sleep and/or REM sleep, the net effect on waking brain information processing (i.e. augmenting versus reducing) would likely depend on which aspects of sleep show relatively greater disruption or attenuation. That is, apnea conditions characterized mainly by deprivation of deep sleep and/or REM sleep *without* phasic REM activity would effect an *increase* in CNS activation during wakefulness relative to pre-morbid levels to help rectify excessively automatized waking attentional processes. This follows because the brain would be deprived of the information-reducing effects of NREM sleep and/or REM sleep unaccompanied by phasic REMS (cf. de la Peña, 1971). Thus, while many apneac individuals may complain of excessive daytime sleepiness, this complaint might be more severe without the presence of the apnea episodes. Other varieties of apnea, characterized more by phasic REM deprivation than NREM sleep (and/or REM sleep without phasic REM activity) deprivation, e.g. deep sleep remains intact, are posited to effect a *reduction* of information processing for the excessively de-automatized brain (infants, some varieties of mental retardation, some varieties of schizophrenia). This is because the apneas effect deprivation of temporal episodes during sleep in which a certain quantity of endogenous sensory information is ordinarily processed.

The posited homeostatic function of certain types of apnea might also explain findings on old age-depression-apnea interrelations. That is, the high degree of automatization of attention characteristic of late and old age might be compensated for to some extent by increments in endogenous sensory information flow during and following apnea periods. McGinty et al (1981) and Smyth et al (1981) have both found that a significant proportion of healthy older males *without* complaint of excessive daytime sleepiness show apneas during sleep which overlap in magnitude with those seen in age-matched patients complaining of excessive daytime sleepiness.

This is not to say that most cases of apnea are to be considered homeostatic and adaptive for the bored waiting brain. Severe chronic cases, wherein there is initiation of life-threatening cardiovascular sequelæ, would represent a *heterostatic* variety of apnea and would be reflective of a generalized disorganization of organismic function (increased systemic entropy) indicative of generalized deautomatization.

THE PARASOMNIAS

Night terrors and nightmares are characterized by abnormally high levels of sensory information flow and/or physiological activation during sleep. My experience with clinic patients suggests that excessive automatization of attention (accompanied by feelings of boredom-anxiety and/or depression) is a primary etiologic element in the genesis of the complaint. The condition is often successfully treated with a stimulating anti-depressant drug (Beitman and Carlin, 1979). I conceptualize the intense barrage of sensory information flow during sleep (in nightmares, very active REM periods; in night terrors, excessive amounts of deep sleep) as compensatory to help rectify the low levels of sensory information flow obtaining during wakefulness and/or sleep as a consequence of excessive attentional automatization.

Enuresis (urination during sleep) is a condition found in children and adults who manifest excessively low levels of physiological activation. It frequently is found in hyperactive boys, and most often is accompanied by a sleep pattern characterized by excessive amounts of deep and REM sleep. The treatment of choice is the anti-depressant medication imipramine. The drug blocks re-uptake of norepinephrine presynaptically, thus enabling more norepinephrine to remain active at the synapse. Enuretic individuals appear to be parasympathetic dominant, i.e., they manifest relatively low levels of physiological activation in most subsystems relative to norms, and are often behaviorally hyperactive (de la Peña, 1980). Imipramine apparently acts to rectify the low levels of sensory information flow during wakefulness and acts to establish a balance in sympathetic and parasympathetic divisions of the nervous system. Since parasympathetic activity increases detrusor muscle contractions and dilates internal sphincters of the bladder, while sympathetic activity effects the opposite changes, the increased sympathetic tone induced by stimulating drugs (and theoretically, long-lasting stimulating information environments) probably accounts for the efficacy of the traditional treatment. I suggest that episodes of nocturnal enuresis may be considered as expressive of a homeostatic sensory information augmenting mechanism which helps to rectify both waking and sleep sensory information underload.[36]

Sleep-walking is another condition for which the same behavioral and physiological correlates obtaining in enuresis apply. The awakenings following nocturnal perambulation might in some instances serve a homeostatic, alerting function and hence rectify a depressed level of sensory information flow during wakefulness, as well as provide a means for awakening an organism that is sleeping too deeply to allow preparation for fight or flight. Sleepwalking, enuresis, and behavioral hyperactivity are often found in the same children and apparently also more often in certain families; this indicates a constitutional predisposition which can be exacerbated by environmental events (depressing conditions, unstimulating environments) which further augment the parasympathetic dominance that lies at the core of automatization of attention.

Finally, I have observed (de la Peña, 1979b) that individuals complaining of headaches, exacerbated or initiated during sleep, frequently show the low physiological activation pattern in most physiological subsystems that is characteristic of enuretics, sleepwalkers, and hyperactive individuals. Imipramine is often an efficacious treatment. In vascular complaints, the etiological mechanism is probably the same as that posited for migraine headache, i.e., excessive dilation of arteries during the periods of profound parasympathetic activity that occurs during sleep. Headaches and the attendant increments in sensory information flow would serve a compensatory sensory augmenting function to rectify aberrantly low levels of information flow during wakefulness or during various stages of sleep, as well as provide an adaptive mechanism to arouse an individual who is too deeply asleep to cope with potentially life-threatening environmental situations and stimuli. Imipramine apparently decreases the amount of vascular dilation, since sympathetic activity acts to constrict blood vessels; as a consequence, the narrowed blood vessels no longer press on surrounding nerves and the pain is alleviated.

Sleep-related gastroesophageal reflux is a disorder in which the individual awakens from sleep either with burning substernal pain, a feeling of general pain or tightness in the chest, or a sour taste in the mouth. Coughing, choking, and vague respiratory discomfort may also be repetitive occurrences with this syndrome (Roffwarg, 1979). While the evidence is not yet conclusive, sleep studies (Welch, 1980) suggest that the problem occurs only during REM sleep, a time of attentional deautomatization. Perhaps the reflex occurs, for the most part, during especially intense REM sleep periods in trophotropic-tuned individuals who are experiencing considerable boredom and depression. In this case, the reflux during sleep is providing compensatory information flow to rectify aberrantly low levels of information flow during wakefulness. In my clinical experience, patients with such complaints show high frequencies of phasic REMs during REM sleep and admit to considerable boredom during wakefulness.

SUMMARY OF SLEEP DISORDERS

Many sleep disorders are apparently associated with excessive automatization of attention during wakefulness and/or sleep. The symptomology, in *acute* cases, apparently provides a compensatory increment in sensory information flow and helps bring the overall sleep-wake sensory information flow into the range that is conducive to organized perceptual-cognitive behavioral function and general adaptation. Nearly always categorized as disorders by the medical establishment and primarily treated by medication, it would seem more reasonable to consider the phenomena, at least in acute cases, along system-organizational, information processing lines and take steps to rectify the excessive automatization of attention which seemingly is a core element in the genesis of the phenomena. Medical intervention would be appropriate when the disorder is chronic and expressive of a generalized heterostatic somatic state, which if uncorrected, will accelerate the demise of the organism.

SEXUAL BEHAVIOR AND GENDER IDENTITY DISORDER

Excessive automatization of attention is apparently of etiological significance in the genesis of certain sexual behavior and gender-identity aberration phenomena.[37] For example, a bored individual may turn to rape, sadism, or masochism in order to rectify feelings of boredom. A bored individual might also seek variety and novelty by adopting the dress, attitudes, and behavior of the opposite sex, as in transvestism and in certain varieties of homosexual behavior.

What is most clear, however, about sexual behavior and sexual aberration is its link with the evolutionary process. That is, sexual reproduction is a relatively new mode of reproduction which came into being only when life achieved a certain degree of complexity and automatization. Asexual reproduction characterized life up to newts and salamanders in phylogeny. It is as if nature reached a certain level of sophistication and automatization, experienced boredom, and subsequently devised a mechanism—sexual reproduction—to expedite the creation of new somatic and psychological genotypes (information).

The sexual act, moreover, provides a very intense state of consciousness which can be used by highly automatized structures to de-automatize consciousness. Finally, one may speculate that the varieties of "aberrations" in gender identity, seemingly more prevalent now than in earlier times (when men were men and women were women) may be reflective, in part, of the trend in evolution for increasing variety and novelty in response to its own increasing and automatization of function.

CONCEPTUALIZATION OF DISORDER, AGING, AND DEATH

An implicit, if not explicit, goal of contemporary medicine is the conquest of disease and the infinite postponement of aging and death. Every day the media provides progress reports from the "war on cancer," "the conquest of disease," etc., as if disease and disorder existed entirely outside of organisms. For example, molecular biologists generally assume that once causative external agents for carcinogenesis and other disease (viruses, chemicals, radiation, etc.) have been identified, they can be eliminated and the war on disease will have been won. This outmoded viewpoint represents carry-over of an obsolete seventeenth century Cartesian dualism into our present world view.

My approach suggests a very different conceptualization of etiology and nature of disease, aging, and death. First, it suggests that there are homeostatic as well as heterostatic aspects of disorder and disease. Literature review pointed out that some varieties of psychological, behavioral, and somatic disorder are clearly homeostatic for brain function, in that they help rectify an excessively automatized consciousness by increasing the information flow for understimulated cognitive structures. That is, some disorders help to de-automatize attention for the excessively automatized brain and thus are commonly observed to result in a higher "personality" integration as the previously excessively bored brain becomes more aware and appreciative of aspects of existence previously taken for granted because of hyperefficient cognitive structures. Other varieties of disorder are clearly heterostatic for existing structures and often reflective of a generalized heterostatic process accruing with old age or conversely, infancy, when cognitive structures are relatively underdeveloped and susceptible to information overload (excessive deautomatization).

Secondly, disease, aging, and death are clearly sequelæ of the evolutionary process and are intimately linked to the development of complexity of structure and automatization of information processing. Phenomena such as depression, pain syndromes, cancer, schizophrenia, ulcers, migraine, cardiovascular disease, etc., are *not* found in organisms *without* nervous systems. The development of life (information) apparently necessitated the invention of disorder and death. Aging, disorder and death, as we recognize it in humans and other animals, did not exist in evolution until the development of diploidy (two chromosomes of each kind) and information processing structures (e. g. a primitive nervous system). Primitive worms, amœba and various one-celled organisms do not age and die; they merely divide or "clone."

With the invention of sexual reproduction, diploidy, aging and death, variety replaced monotony as the basic law of nature. It appears that nature evolved to a point in which a sufficient level of information processing sophistication and automatization obtained for the experience of boredom. Death and sexual reproduction may be the expression of a mechanism whereby nature may replace non-curious, worn-out lower-level structures (cells, organisms) which are unlikely to provide the higher unit (nature) with information, with a new piece of information or consciousness (a new new cell, a new organism) which has more potential for generating information. Thus relatively automatized macro-structures (brain, nature) employ death, disease, and disorder in infra-structures (tissues, individuals) as mechanisms for acceleration of the process of change (information) to levels of information flow conducive to organized function of the macro-structures (Jantsch, 1980).

For the individual organism, aging and death seem to be accelerated by excessive automatization as well as excessive deautomatization of information processing. Anecdotal reports seem consistent with the view that chronic boredom as well as chronic overexcitation accelerate the aging process and death. Overexcitation, presumably associated with deficient cognitive structures for organizing information, probably contributes to the early natural deaths of many mentally retarded individuals. For the vast majority of humankind, however, there is the suggestion that chronic boredom is the primary accelerator of aging and death. The individual who retains a high (but not excessively high) degree of interest and activity in the world with increasing chronological age is the one who apparently best withstands the aging process.

Chronic boredom may accelerate aging and death because understimulated cognitive structures signal the need for processes which change the situation and rectify the boredom. Aging and death both inherently bring *change* and thus information for the bored brain and other supra-structures in the hierarchy of structures in nature.

In this context, total eradication of disorder and disease seems an unworthy goal.   First, if individuals did not die, there would be insufficient planetary resources for survival of most of them. Second, while the elimination of disease would be adaptive for individuals characterized by excessive de-automatization and heterostasis, it might be disastrous for the excessively automatized individual for whom acute illness provides homeostatic stimulation or information. Findings that cancer patients often show *superior* pre-morbid health underscore the possible validity of this viewpoint.   That is, perhaps some individuals develop cancer because they do not normally have access to less lethal forms of information (illness).

The suggestion is that disease and disorder always occur vis-à-vis structures in a hierarchy of structures in nature. What is adaptive or life maintaining for a structure at one level of organization may be maladaptive for other structures at lower or higher levels in the hierarchy of structures in nature.   The current medical viewpoint, which treats health and disease from an exclusively *organismic* viewpoint, is thus considered chauvinistic, anachronistic and obsolete, and perhaps even stultifying to the future evolution of nature.

Chapter 10 Toward a Psychobiology of Health and Disease

The argument that mind-is-only-brain seems logical and solid enough until one remembers that animal life is not merely a collection of biological systems, but is singularly distinguished from the inanimate by an exquisitely harmonious communion among all functional parts, and by elaborate, unifying mutual interdependencies that produce an invisible whole whose qualities transcend the physical elements of its parts.

Barbara Brown
Supermind

INTRODUCTION

The last chapter described the application of mismatch theory to a broad range of somatic and behavioral phenomena. It pointed out the possibility that many health-related phenomena, traditionally viewed by the medical establishment as disorder, may play a homeostatic adaptive role in effecting optimal levels/rates of informational processing for the brain; however, often this occurs at the expense of the integrity of sub- or supra-structures within the hierarchy of organizational structures comprising nature. A major idea of the last chapter is that contemporary models of health and disease are invalid because they have largely ignored the central role of development/evolution in the genesis of contemporary society's most vexing somatic and behavioral disorders. That is, automatization of attentional processes, a legacy or sequela of the evolutionary process, was shown to be intimately associated with a broad spectrum of health-disorder phenomena, including somatic phenomena such as asthma, hypoglycemia, ulcers, cancer, and hypertension, etc; behavioral phenomena such as hyperactivity, violence, gambling, drug abuse, chronic pain syndromes, and schizophrenia; and many sleep disorders. Thus, one achievement of the last chapter is to point out the interrelatedness of many processes which are considered as separate and distinct by contemporary medicine.

A second major idea, more implied than precisely stated in the first few chapters, is that the current medical approach to health and disorder is clearly inefficient with respect to both clinical and research work. This is because the medical model, with its reductionistic, Cartesian spectacles and belief in univariate cause and effect relationships, only permits focus on increasingly minute and trivial parts of the world; and because the reigning assumption that the whole can be understood through a fine analysis of parts, and ultimately the whole can be synthesized from knowledge of its parts, is an anachronistic belief that runs counter to twentieth century science and philosophy. The end result is a narrowness of focus, which is oblivious to interrelations among parts in the hierarchy of structures comprising the universe. The consequence is that modern medicine is characterized by various brands of somatic or psychological chauvinism, and the forest is never seen for the trees. In fact, the trees are rarely seen for the leaves, and the idea that the forest might only be a small but interrelated part of a larger park is not usually entertained. This is not a new idea. It has been articulated by increasing numbers of scientists, health-care practitioners, and health-care critics (Battista, 1977; Moser, 1978; Pelletier, 1978, 1979; Capra, 1979; Bateson, 1979; Toffler, 1980).

A third major idea, primarily outlined in Chapters 2 and 3, is that the beginnings of a more valid epistemology of health phenomena will most likely emerge from the convergence of disciplines such as information and systems theory, cybernetics and control theory, contemporary physics and cognitive psychology. This approach, the world as organization, with an emphasis on developmental and cognitive processes, is at the core of the relatively young holistic approach in medicine. Still in its infancy, the approach shows signs of providing the conceptual foundations for a set of beliefs and practices deserving of the name medicine.

THE ASCENDANCE OF THE SYSTEMS APPROACH IN SCIENTIFIC RESEARCH: THE WORLD AS INFORMATION

Von Bertalanffy has outlined the problems and implications of the systems approach. In biology, behavioral and social science, many phenomena are encountered which are not found in inanimate nature and for which conventional Newtonian physics must remain mute. Von Bertalanffy writes: (1969: 61-63).

> We cannot speak of living things and of behavior except in a functional manner, that is regarding their parts and processes as organized in view of the maintenance, development, evolution, etc., of the system.
> Organismic processes as a rule are so ordered as to maintain the system. But this makes no sense

within the conventional categories of physical and chemical processes taking place in a living organism and those in a corpse; both follow the same laws of physics and chemistry—and that's all that can be said. To the biologist and physician, however, there is a profound difference between events so ordered as to maintain the system, and those running wild to destroy it. What are the principles of order and organization? What does health or norm mean in contrast to disease and pathology? Nothing, so far as laws of physics and chemistry are concerned and mechanistic philosophy is adopted. But without these and similar notions there would be no science of medicine and indeed of biology . . . . In summary: There are recent developments, loosely circumscribed by the concept of system, which try to answer the demands mentioned. In contrast to the progressive and necessary specialization of modern science, they let us hope for a new integration and conceptual organization. Speaking in terms of natural philosophy, as against the world as chaos, a new conception of the world as organization seems to emerge.

He continues (1969: 70-71):

General system theory may be considered a science of wholeness or holistic entities which hitherto, that is, under the mechanistic bias, were excluded as unscientific, vitalistic or metaphysical. Within the framework of general systems theory these aspects become scientifically accessible. General system, therefore, is an interdisciplinary model which needs, but also is capable of, scientific elaboration and consequently can be applied to concrete phenomena. This is its "scientific" aspect. Like every more general theory or model, it also has its aspects as "metascience" or "natural philosophy"; that is, it influences our world outlook, and appears to be broader and more realistic than previous, mechanistic philosophy.

If at present general system theory is capable of dealing, in exact terms, with only a limited range of phenomena, while many others can be dealt with only in more or less loose verbal language or not at all, it is well to remember the history of science. Galileo's and Newton's universes were but a minute fraction of the physical world known to nineteeth-century physics, which in turn has increased immeasurably during our lifetime. Perhaps more precisely: System theory probably is in a phase comparable to electrodynamics at the time of Faraday and before Maxwell; principles are intuitively seen, but a genius is needed to provide mathematical theory.[38]

A Holistic Conceptualization of Health and Disease

Literature review in the previous chapter offers suggestions for some first steps in the construction of a systems conceptualization of health and disease. It is suggested that the terms may be more validly couched in terms of order and disorder, information and entropy. One tentative conclusion is that each successive level of organization in nature—from fundamental particles in physics to biological organisms to collections of biological organisms—may have an optimal level of information processing for organized function and general viability. Health or order obtains when the amount of information processed from the environment by a given structural unit remains within some optimal range for organized function of the unit. Growth or development occurs when the optimal range of information processing of an organizational unit is exceeded or undershot (mismatch is experienced) for a period of time which is not so excessive that existing structures are irreparably damaged, but which persists long enough to allow the creation of new structures which can better deal with the information overload or underload stress. Disease or disorder obtains when there is a sufficiently intense and/or persistent mismatch between a given structural unit's information organizing capacity and the amount of information processed from the structure's environment, such that the organization unit shows disorganized function and/or irreparable breakdown.

As noted in Chapter 2, a basic premise of my approach is that the higher the organizational unit in the hierarchy of organizational units in nature, the greater the information organizing capacity and the amount of information needed for optimal function and continued integrity of the unit. All of the units of organization in nature are presumed to experience varying degrees of match or mismatch of optimal information load at various points in time. However, it appears that prioritizing of rectification of mismatch operates in hierarchical fashion, with higher level organization units having priority over lower level units with respect to effecting optimal information processing loads. For example, when the brain experiences a match between optimal and de facto information processing loads it acts as a beneficent health care provider (cf. Schwartz, 1977) for lower level structures experiencing mismatch (e.g., indigestion in the stomach), coordinating a complex pattern of autonomic, skeletal muscle, and sensory controls to keep information flow within optimal range for the structure (stomach) experiencing mismatch. That is, there is some suggestion that the brain performs its role as healer (to use Pelletier's term) to the extent that it is experiencing a rate and/or amount of information flow that is within its optimal range for organized function.

When the brain is experiencing significant *mismatch* however, it appears that mind is more slayer than healer (Pelletier's descriptors). For example, an understimulated, bored brain may initiate a pattern of autonomic, skeletal muscle, cortical and sensory controls (e.g., smoking cigarettes or drinking alcohol excessively, hallucinating, creating delusions, engaging in risky behaviors) which may ultimately result in the demise of substructures such as lung, liver, or supra-structures such as the body, or family (from gambling, violent behavior, etc.).

This view of nature will no doubt seem strange, foreign and perhaps even unpalatable to establishment science, medicine, and psychology. A core concept is the premise that mind or intelligence is ubiquitous in nature and not confined to the brain and/or central nervous system of homo sapiens. The premise is at the heart of most systems approaches to nature and one that is being voiced by growing numbers of the world's most brilliant thinkers in the fields of contemporary physics (Walker, 1970; Sarfatti, 1975; Bohm, 1980); philosophy (Butler, 1924; de Chardin, 1950; von Bertalanffy, 1967; Bateson, 1979); biology (Jantsch, 1980); and contemporary psychology (Globus, 1976; John, 1976; Battista, 1979; Brown, 1980).[39]

The Concept of Behavioral Medicine

The holistic systems approach is finally encroaching upon the fields of medicine and psychology. The recent emergence of concepts such as behavioral medicine, holistic health and health psychology, are testimony to this growing trend. Behavioral medicine is a comparatively new field of inquiry and practice. While it lies at the interface between traditional clinical psychology, physiological psychology, psychiatry, and medicine, its metaphysics, epistemology and general premises about the nature of health and disease, the mind-body problem, etc., are sufficiently different from the traditional fields that it is generally considered a revisionist movement within behavioral science.

Schwartz and Weiss (1978) define the field thus:

> Behavioral medicine is the interdisciplinary field concerned with the development and integration of behavioral and biomedical science, knowledge, and techniques relevant to health and illness and the application of this knowledge and these techniques to prevention, diagnosis, treatment and rehabilitation.

Schwartz and Weiss elaborate:

> We believe that this shift in emphasis reflects

more than semantics. It reflects an important change in conceptualization, in which traditional mental vs. physical disorders are no longer described in purely behavioral vs. biological terms, but rather are conceived and studied from a more integrated, biobehavioral perspective. This shift in orientation may well represent a shift in paradigm (Kuhn, 1962), one that will, in the long run, have significant implications for all aspects of theory, research, and applications involving health and illness. It certainly reflects a challenge for future research, establishing the requirement for continued development of interdisciplinary thinking and research as the *sine qua non* for this field.

THE RE-ASCENDANCE OF CONSCIOUSNESS AS THE CENTRAL PROBLEM IN PHYSICAL AND BEHAVIORAL SCIENCE

Consciousness in the Physical Sciences

It appears that psychologists are not the only ones to recognize the central role of consciousness in behavior. Laymen, logicians, and the physical scientists have joined the parade. In the field of logic, for example, Kurt Godel's Incompleteness Theorem [40] presented formal proof of a nonlogical component in all logical systems. The implication, with one reservation in mind,[41] is that any comprehensive inquiry into the nature of consciousness must be incomplete if based purely upon logical information.

Nowhere in physical science is the emergence of consciousness more prominent than in contemporary physics. At present, there is great controversy in contemporary physics about the nature of physical reality and its interrelation with consciousness. The first physicist to undermine the old notions of reality was Werner Heisenberg. His uncertainty principle states that the position and momentum of an atomic particle are complementary quantities that can only be approximated, not precisely known. That is, as physicists attempt to measure one variable with greater precision, the value of the other becomes more uncertain. That the uncertainty is not simply a matter of the physical limitations of present instruments was conclusively demonstrated.[42]

The philosophical implications of the uncertainty principle mark the limits of any and all strictly deterministic interpretations of the physical universe (Pelletier, 1978). A strictly deterministic paradigm requires that an observer be capable of ascertaining the position and momentum of even the most elementary particles. Heisenberg's demonstration of the impossibility of such observations (the very act of measurement or observation transmits sufficient energy to alter the observed system) points out the necessity of acknowledging the nonobjective components of any comprehensive system of inquiry.

Heisenberg's uncertainty principle has profound implications for the study of consciousness. Since all other sciences are based upon models derived from the natural sciences, especially physics, the implication is that research into the nature of consciousness cannot validly employ the old paradigms. Moreover, the principle points out the limit imposed on the accuracy of knowledge about individual entities. Only average values of a great many single observations can be predicted with any degree of accuracy. Averaging procedures performed on multiple events lie at the base of quantum theory, while quantum mechanics describes systems in statistical terms that generate the probability of a particular outcome. Finally, physicists find it increasingly necessary to refer to subatomic, nonobservable entities. Descriptions of the characteristics of these invisible particles and of their governing processes sound remarkably similar to properties that psychology ascribes to the phenomena of consciousness (e.g., tachyons, charm, quarks, virtual particles).

Of late, other physicists have contributed hypotheses about the nature of reality. Theorists such as Popper (1956) argue for the existence of a single, objective reality, while others such as Everett (1957) argue for the existence of multiple simultaneous realities. Walker (1972) speculates that photons may be conscious.

> Consciousness may be associated with all quantum mechanical processes . . . since everything that occurs is ultimately the result of one or more quantum mechanical events, the universe is inhabited by an almost unlimited number of rather discrete conscious, usually nonthinking entities that are responsible for the detailed working of the universe.

Wigner (1972) contends that consciousness causes physical reality to take on a particular form; his contention is supported by the empirical verification of Bell's theorem[43] (Stapp, 1975) which indicates the existence of nonlocal causality (faster-than-light information transfer) and implies that how a physicist decides to do an experiment may partially determine the result found by another physicist in a spatially disconnected part of the universe. Stapp (1975) suggests that we can never understand the ultimate nature of physical reality but must content ourselves with hypotheses about how such reality is revealed to us.

The Return of Consciousness to Psychology

Growing numbers of eminent establishment psychologists are emphasizing the central place of consciousness in psychological science. The psychologist Ernest Hilgard has recently provided historical perspective for the re-emergence of consciousness in contemporary psychology (Hilgard, 1980). In addition he describes how many topical areas in psychology have become cognitive in orientation, e.g., developmental psychology, psycholinguistics, sleep and dreams, psychopharmacology, social psychology, personality, hypnosis, clinical psychology, humanistic and transpersonal psychology.   The neuropsychologist E. Roy John (1976) defines consciousness as an emergent property of sufficiently complex matter.   Karl Pribram's constructional realism model of consciousness (Pribram, 1976) employs hologram theory models to suggest how consciousness is derived from the physical structure of the brain.   The psychobiologist Roger Sperry (1977: 237) summarizes his position:

> The traditional dichotomy that has separated science and value judgement and set corresponding limitations to the domain and role of science is challenged in the context of recent developments in the concept of consciousness and mind-brain relations. A conceptual explanatory model for psychophysical interaction has emerged during the past decade that changes the scientific status of subjective experience and negates many mechanistic, deterministic, and reductionistic features of prior materialist-behavioral doctrine.   Subjective values, conceived in the present terms, transcend their neural components in brain function to become causal determinants per se with objective consequences.   The strategic control power of human values functioning as universal cerebral determinants in all social decision making is emphasized, along with logical indications for a more active involvement therein on the part of science.

In my opinion, the most comprehensive and valid theory of consciousness to date has been formulated by the psychiatrist John Battista (1978: 83).   His information holism model clearly takes into account developmental, hierarchical factors. After reviewing a broad range of literature in psychology and physics, he concludes:

> Information holism also has a number of exciting implications for the nature of reality.   First, reality is neither singular nor objective. Rather, the universe is a unified whole that is hierarchically ordered into different levels of reality, each referring to a particular level of information. Information is inherently relational and involves the interaction of two structures, one serving as the source of data and the other as the receiver. Information is neither subjective nor objective. Subjectivity and objectivity refer to the relative hierarchical relationship between two interacting structures.   A

lower-level structure will appear objective, the structure interacting with that lower level will be experienced subjectively.

Thus, informational holism is holistic. It is neither dualistic nor monistic. Both dualism and monism are accepted as aspects of an integrated and unified system. There is no mind-body problem. Mind and body refer to different hierarchical levels of the same unified system. Many readers will recognize the relationship between informational holism and general system theory. In fact informational holism is based on the holistic paradigm that underlies general system theory (Battista, 1977). Informational holism can thus be considered to be a part of a unified general system theory of the universe.

Unlike his counterpart E. Hilgard (1980), who urges restraint and conservatism in theorizing about ultimate questions, Battista makes some bold, yet careful, conceptual thrusts into such matters (Battista, 1978: 83-84):

An even more interesting prediction emerges from applying informational holism to objects such as groups and institutes that transcend traditional physical boundaries and are defined by their information-processing structures. Informational holism would clearly predict that groups have consciousness, thus giving credence to thinking of the mind and vitality of social organizations.

From my own perspective, the most interesting prediction of informational holism comes from attempting to apply it to the universe as a whole. It is impossible to develop a complete understanding of the universe as a whole because each individual is a part of it and any attempt to understand it will modify it. However, even given this limitation it is quite clear that it would make sense to talk about a seventh level of information that would involve the universe's experience as a whole and refer to the interaction and coordination of all the lower levels of information. The implications of informational holism for spirituality and transpersonal consciousness is thus a very exciting area for further investigation.

Similar ideas have been published by the psychiatrist G. Globus (1974) and the philosopher A. M. Young (1976).

A SUMMARY OF THE BOOK

Colin Wilson has written a stunning series of books about the contemporary predicament of man; for Wilson, evolution is a two-edged proposition. At one edge, increments in experience give man unparalleled ability among other forms in nature to analyze and focus the environment into parts so that he is better able to organize, model, and predict the blooming, buzzing confusion that is reality. Thus, man is generally considered to be the most intelligent, sophisticated and adaptable of all varieties of organization in nature.

However, Wilson contends that by virtue of the same abilities man employs to analyze, dissect, and focus the environment, man is left in "a low intensity of consciousness." That is, what we label intelligence might just as legitimately be labeled "tunnel vision," "the worm's eye view" or "narrowness of perception." Owing to man's great ability to focus, analyze and categorize experience, he is left with only a small trickle of the possible reality coming through the reducing valve or filter of cognitive processes. The result is boredom, a sense of futility and depression in day-to-day encounters with ordinary environments.

In order to escape the "triviality of everydayness," man invented the arts and sciences, since these allow the perception of wider, novel and more dramatic vistas. On the other hand, many of man's greatest problems and threats to the existence on the planet—alcoholism, war, violence, paranoia, schizophrenia, risk-taking—are viewed as compensatory attempts by the evolved, experienced and bored brain to augment the intensity of consciousness to levels which are associated with feeling more alive, experiencing "meaning" and a unitive state of consciousness with the universe.

When I first chanced upon Wilson's work in 1972, I had independently come to many of the same conclusions. My dissertation, "The Psychobiology of the Rapid Eye Movement Dream State" (1971), put forth hypotheses about interrelations of increments in experience with phenomena such as REM sleep, waking perception, schizophrenia, hyperactivity, violence, and hypersexuality. Increments in experience were posited to be associated with a narrowing of the beam of attention and with subsequent cortical efforts to rectify the information deprivation. Reading Wilson for the first time was like reading my own work, except that his was written in a highly artistic, elegant style which used the novel as the primary vehicle of communication. Wilson's ideas and works reinforced my thinking about the structure of nature and served a unique booster function for my perception of nature.

About a year later, after having read much on the psychobiology of cancer, it occurred to me that cancer was yet another phenomenon to which our general framework had application. The result was the formulation of the hypotheses which are described in Chapters 4-7 of this book. About two years after completion of the first draft of this book, I began to realize that our general theoretical constructs had broader applicability to many other health related phenomena. The result is Chapters 8 and 9.

Finally, in the last few years I have been trying to keep abreast of developments in contemporary cognitive psychology and physics and I have been impressed by the gradual dissolution of the boundaries between these disciplines. Implications of the confluence of psychology and physics form the bulk of this last chapter.

THE CRITICAL NEED FOR A VALID EPISTEMOLOGY OF NATURE

Nature at the Crossroads in Its Evolution

The decade of the seventies has abounded in apocalyptic predictions about the future of man. Daily the media bombard us with images and words about economic problems, disintegration of the family structure, environmental pollution, the weakening of the church, increased rates of boredom and suicide, fragmentation of knowledge into highly specialized compartments, the threat of nuclear annihilation, etc. Indeed, the gloomy, pessimistic prognosis for the future of nature is seemingly shared, at first glance, by mismatch theory. For example, if the mismatch hypothesis has validity at supra-levels of structure in nature (cities, states, countries, nations), it may be in the order of things in the developed countries that peace will be short-lived as evolution continues along its steady course. This is because there will be more and more need for war and/or competition at various levels of behavior (verbal, physical, intellectual) among these larger units because the more experienced and/or evolved the unit, the higher the need for information and/or stimulation for organized function of the unit. Certainly this conforms to the unsophisticated viewpoint of even the most casual of observers of the global condition, i.e., order and harmony between individuals, cities, states, countries, etc., seem decidedly short-lived.

In the face of this apparent chain of rapid individual, social and ecological change, is another strongly enunciated viewpoint which views upheaval as symptomatic of a profound evolutionary transformation of human consciousness (Pelletier, 1979; Toffler, 1980). For this group, the dismal predictions of future society (population glut, little or no freedom for individual expression, the linear progression to nuclear destruction) are viewed as events marking the end of an outmoded conception of the individual and his most fundamental beliefs. A fundamental re-orientation of modern man's world view is involved: rather than viewing himself and his environment as a fragmented cosmic machine, the new viewpoint stresses the interdependence of organism and environment. This is the *perspectivist* philosophy now emerging in psychology, physics and in some sectors of modern medicine.[44]   The physicist Werner Heisenberg eloquently states in *Across the Frontier* (1974: 68):

> A feeling will gradually grow up that life on
> earth represents a unity, that damage at one point
> can have effects everywhere else, that we are
> jointly responsible for the ordering of life upon this
> our earth. From the cosmic distances to which man
> can penetrate by means of modern technology, we
> see perhaps more clearly than from earth itself the
> unitary laws whereby all life on our planet is order-
> ed.

Secondly, a major change in paradigm has to do with the nature of
consciousness. The old metaphysics and epistemology assume that
consciousness and information processing is a *passive* phenomenon,
i.e., our perceptions are more or less a passive reflection of some
external and internal reality. The current viewpoint is illustrated in a
quote taken from a recent article (Trillin, 1981: 701) written by a
woman who had undergone a pulmonary lobectomy for adenocarcinoma
of the lung at the age of thirty-eight.

> It astonishes me that having faced the terror, we
> continue to live, even to live with a great deal of
> joy. It is commonplace for people who have can-
> cer—particularly those who feel as well as I do—to
> talk about how much richer their lives are because
> they have confronted death. Yes, my life is very
> rich. I have even begun to understand that wonder-
> ful line in *King Lear*, "Ripeness is all." I suppose
> that becoming ripe means finding out that none of
> the really important questions have answers. I wish
> that life had devised a less terrifying, less risky way
> of making me ripe. *But I wasn't given any choice
> about this.* [Emphasis in original.]

Trillin's viewpoint has been obliterated in the last decade by a barrage
of studies in psychology and contemporary physics. The new view
posits consciousness as an active, organizing, principle that coordin-
ates the divergent functions of the physical brain in an organized
manner and which operates at the quantum level where "mind" and
"matter" are in inextricable interaction (Pelletier, 1978; Sperry, 1976).

The views expressed in this book support the emerging holistic
viewpoint. A fundamental premise is that consciousness is a variable
which can be controlled by units of organization "from within."
Evolving organisms are not necessarily locked into an ever-escalating
"homeostatic" cognitive, somatic, and behavioral hyperactivity (violence, aggression, cancer, etc.) due to increasing automatization and
the subsequent functional information underload. Rather, the suggestion is that highly sophisticated brains can learn methods and/or
techniques of de-automatization so that they can see the familiar as
strange or the universe in a grain of sand (Ornstein, 1972). This is the

next step in the evolution of nature; such a creature will be able to match his information organizing capacity to best fit environmental demands. He will not allow himself to experience boredom (information underload) or overexcitement (information overload) for very long unless he so desires. That is, he will enjoy an enlarged capacity for self-regulation and entertainment. This needs to occur in larger proportions of the population (isolated individuals with high capacities for self-entertainment already exist to be sure); nothing less than planetary survival hinges on the realization of this goal (Bateson, 1972; 1979).

Toward a Psychobiology of Health and Disease

Progress toward a comprehensive, valid viewpoint of health and disease can no longer ignore psycho-social factors and consciousness in the etiology of health and disease. In fact, more knowledge about the nature of consciousness, *and the role of the unconscious* (Shevrin and Dickman, 1980), seems critical for the future development of a true science of health and disease. In my opinion, man is at a curious point in his evolution. On the one hand, the majority of men are still not quite human, the triviality of everydayness eats away at their psyches and produces a host of behavioral, cognitive and physical disorders, sometimes culminating in death. On the other hand, a handful of thinkers around the world seem to be on the verge of achieving a unified field theory of nature which greatly surpasses in scope and implications the unified field theory that eluded Einstein and continues to baffle his successors. For the first time in the history of nature, nature is close to the point where it is now possible to outline hypotheses about itself wherein the student of life science may perceive the unity and underlying threads connecting all of its parts.

The construct of consciousness is the key to these endeavors. At present, physics considers four fundamental forces to account for all known phenomena: (1) electromagnetic forces, which deal with medium scale phenomena and are most applicable in addressing living organisms; (2) gravity, which accounts for interactions between very large bodies ranging from ordinary objects to solar systems and galaxies; (3) weak nuclear force; and (4) strong nuclear force—both of which account for phenomena at the infinitesimal levels of subatomic physics. Despite the considerable explanatory power of these four forces, a growing number of contemporary physicists seem predisposed to posit at least one more force to account for certain inexplicable phenomena occurring below the limits of instrumental observation. This factor is consciousness or information (Sarfatti, 1975; Capra, 1975; Stapp, 1975).

Contemporary physics is thus on the verge of being transformed from the study of forces interacting with inert objects to a science which studies the dynamic properties of living conscious systems since even the smallest parts of nature appear to have consciousness to some degree.

Perhaps the situation is the other way around and physics will be gradually subsumed under psychology. This is Piaget's view (1979). He writes (1978: 648):

> Five points are made: (1) Psychology is the science not only of the individual but also of humans in general. For example, mathematics and physics have been created by human beings, and this creation can be understood only in terms of human intelligence in its totality. (2) Psychology is a natural science, and, like every other science, it is built not only with what comes from the object but also with the structures constructed by the subject. (3) Psychology occupies a key position among the sciences because it explains the notions and operations used in the development of all the sciences. (4) It is impossible to dissociate psychology from epistemology. (5) Psychology, like all other sciences, can thrive only on interdisciplinary cooperation.

Another perspective concerning the establishment of a science of consciousness points out the central role of psychology. Wigner (1970: 37) writes:

> That a higher integration of science is needed is perhaps best demonstrated by the observation that the basic entities of intuitionistic mathematics are the physical objects, that the basic concept in the epistemological structure of physics is the concept of observation, and that psychology is not yet ready for providing concepts and idealizations of such precision as are expected in mathematics or even physics. Thus this passing of responsibility from mathematics to physics, and hence to the science of cognition, ends nowhere. This state of affairs should be remedied by a closer integration of the now separate disciplines.

This book provides a very rough approximation of a new metaphysics and epistemology which may form the bedrock of future conceptualizations of the psychobiology of health and disease. Its key ideas are the world and consciousness as organization or information; the hierarchical, developmental structure of nature; and the interrelatedness of all parts comprising nature, where the parts are seen to be arbitrary constrictions of our unique psychobiological heritage and endowment (von Bertalanffy, 1969; Dewan, 1976; Bohm, 1980).

What is needed more than ever before in the history of nature is a valid paradigm from which to study nature. This paradigm must provide a more valid metaphysics and epistemology than currently exists. This suggests a revolution in the techniques, paradigm, and methodology of research endeavors,[45] indeed the very style,[46] of inquiry. The emerging holistic paradigm seems best suited to serve as the building block for a valid metatheoretical foundation for science. It shows promise of providing valid definitions and conceptions of the mind-body problem, medicine and psychosomatic medicine, consciousness and personality, health and disease, the aging process, stress, life, and death. This knowledge will ultimately accelerate the evolution and self-actualization of nature. To quote Wilson once more (1979: 630):

> Human beings will one day recognize beyond all possibility of doubt that consciousness is freedom. When this happens consciousness will cease to suffer from mistrust of its own nature. Suddenly the profits will be clear and self-evident. Instead of wasting most of its energies in retreats and uncertainties and excursions into blind alleys, consciousness will recycle its energies into its own evolution. The feedback point will mark a new stage in the history of the planet earth. When that happens, the first fully human being will be born.

Notes

[1] Physical reactions vary from augmented metastatic responses to instances of "spontaneous remission," where ostensibly terminal cancer is halted in its progress or disappears completely. Cancer, with its threat of impending death, apparently may act to rekindle an appreciation of aspects of life which had previously come to be taken for granted, one's own integrity, friends, the amazing variety of nature, etc. The writer Susan Sontag described this effect in a television interview with Dick Cavett. When queried by Cavett about her feelings during the time when her cancer was in apparent remission, she stated that in some sense she missed the feeling of emergency and crisis associated with the initial diagnosis, since the threat of death resulted in her regaining appreciation of many aspects of her life which she had come to take for granted. Now with the cancer gradually regressing, she sensed herself slipping back into her previous robotic state of existence. The journalist Stewart Alsop, in *Stay of Execution* (1973) wrote the following about his struggle with cancer: "In a way, no experience has been more interesting than living in intermittent intimacy with the gentleman W. C. Fields used to call 'the man in the white nightgown' . . . . Death is, after all, the only universal experience except birth, and although a sensible person hopes to put it off as long as possible, it is, even in anticipation, an interesting experience."

[2] Other evidence for primitivity of function in tumor cells is suggested from studies of oxygen deprivation. One characteristic of tumor cells is their ability to remain viable for as long as three days in an environment containing cyanide and totally lacking in oxygen (Warburg, 1926). In contrast, normal cells die within minutes when exposed to the same environment. Similarly, at the organism level, the human newborn is remarkably resistant to oxygen-lack relative to human adults (Richter, 1961). Anærobic metabolism (glycolysis) is phylogenetically a more primitive mode of energy production than ærobic "respiration," e.g., metabolism in the more evolved vertebrates involves the utilization of oxygen, and metabolism in less evolved bacteria is completely

anaerobic.

3

Chemical carcinogenesis is generally a two-stage process, initiation, followed by promotion. Croton oil alone rarely produces skin cancer, but if a polycyclic hydrocarbon is applied to the skin of an experimental animal, and croton oil is then applied, skin cancer frequently occurs. In this case, the polycyclic hydrocarbon acts as an initiator and the croton oil as a promotor.

4

The relation between disorganization and information processing is described in detail in the section outlining the premises of the developmental-structural approach.

5

For a more formal explanation of the concepts of information and entropy, see Gatlin (1972).

6

It is not possible to specify, with any certainty, the detailed neural organization of this regulating mechanism. It is possible that the level of physiological activation (i.e., the information processing rate) is monitored either via a polysensory system, like the reticular formation, or through detection of an electrical correlate of the level of processing such as d.c. potential changes.

7

Powers' (1973) contribution is the latest and perhaps the most incisive synthesis and commentary on applying the concept of feedback-control systems to brain organization and the psychology of perception. His main thesis is that our perceptions are the only reality we can know, and that the purpose of all our actions is to control the state of this perceived world.

8

The notion of cholinergic dominance during NREM sleep can account for this apparent exception. The transmitter agent at all ganglionic synapses in both the sympathetic and parasympathetic divisions of the autonomic nervous system is acetylcholine (ACH). ACH is the transmitter at the postganglionic neuroeffector synapses of the parasympathetic system while norepinephrine is the transmitter of postganglionic neuroeffector synapses of the sympathetic system. Sweat gland activity (GSR) is the one exception to this rule: sympathetic postganglionic innervation of the sweat glands is mediated by ACH (1967).

9

Furst (1979: 91-92) writes: As in the case with many matters of subjective experience, the psychologist's understanding of automatizing has been anticipated by that of writers and poets. In slightly different language, the notion of auto-

maticity in perception has been a recurrent theme in literature. Romantic poets have dwelt on the lost innocence of
childhood, a time when we once perceived things with greater
awareness. William Wordsworth wrote:

> There was a time when meadow, grove and
> stream,
> The earth and every common sight,
> To me did seem
> Apparelled in celestial light,
> The glory and the freshness of a dream.

Henry David Thoreau (1817-1863), associated with the
romantic period in American literature, talked about the
trick of bending over to look at the world between his legs.
Inverting the visual field in this way produces a curious
strangeness to familiar objects. You might try this for
yourself, when no one is watching.

All this can be translated into our terms: a child, lacking
in experience, has not developed the cognitive structure
which would let him process visual information less intensely.
And Thoreau, looking between his legs, is carrying out an
operation analogous to dis-habituation.

10 In studies of normal subjects, the maintenance of a perceptually undifferentiated orientation to stimulation has been
shown to be associated with a greater sensitivity to low
intensity stimulation than is the maintenance of an analyti-
cally differentiated set to stimulation (Allison, 1963; Kaswan
et al, 1965).

11 For a formal explication of this problem, see Kacser (1957:
231-233).

12 The SSS consists of thirty-four forced-choice item pairs,
developed on the basis of factor analysis, describing a stimulating and a less stimulating activity of each pair. A number
of theoretically predicted relationships between the SSS
score and other measures have been empirically confirmed
and thus provide some degree of construct validity for the
scale (Farley and Farley, 1967; Zuckerman, 1974).

13 One implication is that some cross-level differences in information processing and control may exist. Miller (1960), in
studies comparing cells, organs, organisms, groups, and organizations, found not only comparable information input-
output functions and adjustment processes (omissions, errors,
queuing, chunking, filtering, abstracting, etc.) across levels,
but also some systematic cross-level differences.

14

The Laws of Newton were adequate in dealing with the interactions of macroscopic bodies, but when Bohr attempted to use them in constructing his model of the atom, the results were quite disappointing, particularly in the quantitative explanation of spectra.

15

Although the claim that the whole is "more than" and "different from" the sum of its parts is usually meant in the sense that the whole cannot be reduced to its parts and their relational properties, Wimsatt (1976) suggests that such a reduction is possible, when "reduction" is properly understood.

16

There is a general consistency in stressor methodology employed in the few Russian investigations which specify details of methodology.

17

Lewis suggested that cancer was a form of paranoia at the cellular level.

18

Freud's (1917) notions on psychodynamic mechanisms in depression dovetail nicely with these suggestions. He conceptualized depression resulting from personal losses of significant others as a turning of part of the self into the lost object. In carcinogenesis, the depressive process is somatized; part of the body is turned into the lost object by way of the neoplastic process, specifically the organ involved biologically or symbolically in the lost object-person relationship.

19

The section thus provides support for the general system theorist position that important formal identities of large generality exist across "levels" of structure.

20

Milk secretion involves the synthesis within the alveolar cells of milk and the subsequent excretion of milk into the alveolar lumen; milk removal concerns the transfer of milk from the alveoli and fine ducts into the large ducts, gland cistern or sinus.

21

Major differences between tobacco smoke and general air pollutants are the particle size and the amount inhaled each day (Hoffman and Wynder, 1968; Wynder and Hoffman, 1972). The cigarette smoker who inhales ingests up to five billion particles per cubic centimeter of smoke. The respiratory defense mechanism is hardly capable of adequate removal of such a dense aerosol, especially since cigarette smoke contains high concentrations of ciliatoxic and mucus-coagulating agents as well. By breathing even heavily polluted air, a person will inhale a maximum of 100,000 particles per cubic centimeter of air.

22   The rate of information processing for the lung might be defined as the rate at which the lungs oxygenate the blood and eliminate carbon dioxide. This capacity would vary directly with development of lung structure. Since the male lung has a greater information-processing capacity relative to the typical female lung, the fact that the incidence of lung cancer in males has risen to epidemic proportions in the past thirty years may in part reflect increments in information underload. This is because increasing numbers of men have assumed sedentary jobs and automation in travel has reduced the opportunity for physical activity (and associated lungular information processing) during the same three decades.

23   The epidemiological findings (Suss et al, 1973) which point out the remarkable connection between social class and stomach cancer would be explained as the effect of poverty on the ability to buy and eat a diet consisting of varied elements (protein, carbohydrates, fats, etc.) The diet of the poor is likely to be informationally poor for the stomach. An alternative explanation is that carbohydrates are associated with information underload because carbohydrates have a much lower stimulating effect on gastric acid secretion than do proteins (Saint-Hilaire et al, 1960).

24   According to Fox (1978), the interval from induction of carcinogenesis to clinical detection (i.e., the latent period) is variable, but can be estimated from observed doubling lives of tumors and doubling times of in-vitro clones. Fox suggests that five years is a good conservative estimate: Peller (1976), going through comparable arguments, suggests a seven year latent period. For breast cancer, Rush (1975) computes an eleven year latent period. For lung cancer, a period of 2.4 years is computed, but since the frequency distribution is strongly skewed to longer times, the average time is meaningfully longer (Fox 1978). These considerations lead to the conclusion that mis-match events taking place during the preceding two or three years are likely irrelevant to cancer induction. Psychological and/or stress factors occurring a few years prior to the manifestation of the carcinogenic process relate more to promotion than to initiation. If both recent and more remote events are included in a retrospective case-control comparison, conclusions about their effect will refer to a mixed bag of cause and growth. Thus, in performing a retrospective study, it is important to attempt to define and differentiate time frames as precisely as possible, e.g., in assessing the variable of interest, one should demarcate later from earlier events and dispositions (e.g.,

one should derive the theoretical latent period from a given tumor type, and use the interval in the construction of the data collection methods and in the analysis and interpretation).

25

Psychophysiological studies suggest that increasing age is associated with decreased physiological activation in most somatic systems of the body; e.g., decreases in pupillary diameter (Weale, 1961), skin conductance, mean frequency of the resting EEG, and heart rate as well as heart rate variability (Steinschneider et al, 1966). Blood pressure is one variable which shows increases with age; recent psychophysiological literature, however, points out that increases in blood pressure may effect decreases in cognitive, ideational information processing.

26

Wishner's (1955) concept of efficiency may lend itself to conceptualizing individual differences in CNS activation, as might the notion of "biologic noise" described by Buss (1966: 345). The mismatch hypothesis posits that the predisposition to develop cancer in adults is most often associated with a high level of CNS efficiency and/or an extremely low level of biological noise.

27

A new bent of the immunological deficiency hypothesis of carcinogenesis—generally referred to by the term "immunosurveillance"—postulates that the majority of tumor cells, induced by physical or chemical carcinogens, or oncogenic viruses, are destroyed or at least kept in check by the tumor specific antigens which they produce, and that only those tumor cells which escape such immunosurveillance cause the development of progressively growing tumors (Good and Finstad, 1969; cf. Burnet, 1968). However, the hypothesis requires certain basic conditions to be satisfied, for which there is little, if any, supporting evidence (cf. Prehn, 1968).

28

However, it is clear that not all forms of carcinogenesis are thus affected (Della Porta et al, 1970; Haran-Ghera and Lurie, 1971) while spontaneous tumors seem hardly affected (Baldwin et al, 1967). Moreover, since neoplastic transformation can occur in vitro, where neither thymectomy or anti-lymphocytic factors are involved, these results cannot, by themselves, serve as proof that neoplastic transformation is essentially an immunological process, even though a change in the immune response of the animal can sometimes influence the overall neoplastic response in vivo (Berenblum, 1974).

29

Studies of interrelations between cancer and physiological activation (Clemens, 1954; Thomas and Greenstreet, 1973;

Selye, 1950), perception (George, 1970), and sleep-dream variables (Abse et al, 1974; Lester et al, 1969) are generally retrospective and "pilot" in nature. There is a great need for prospective, systematic resarch in this area.

30 Ordinarily, high development of cortical structure (particularly frontal cortex structure), high sensory thresholds, and low levels of physiological activation go together (cf. de la Peña, 1971).

31 The writer interprets the present jogging phenomenon and the general ascendance of participatory sports as a compensatory response to the automatization of attentional processes that afflicts most individuals in our highly evolved contemporary Western society. That is, one jogs or attends sporting events, in part, to de-automatize excessively automatized attentional processes.

32 For an excellent review and typology of cognitive-behavioral techniques used to rectify mismatch of optimal information load, see Davidson and Schwartz's chapter on the psychobiology of relaxation (1976).

33 The theoretical rationale for positing mind as an inherent property of larger organizational units such as corporation, state, country, nation, etc., is outlined in a chapter on the mind-body problem appearing in the sequel to this book. In the sequel, I review a broad range of literature from contemporary neuropsychology, cognitive psychology and physics which supports the notion of "mind" as an emergent property of sufficiently complex and appropriately organized matter and as ubiquitous and hierarchically organized in nature.

34 Drawing upon current knowledge in modern biology; developmental, introspective and social psychology; cultural anthropology; psychopathology and psychiatry; linguistics; history of culture, etc., von Bertalanffy (1964) has concluded that the traditional Cartesian dualism of mind and body cannot be maintained either with respect to immediate experience or to the constructs of physics and psychology.

35 Competition probably exists between the various levels of organizational units in effecting an optimal range of information processing for themselves. It is probable that suprastructures or supra-units of organization control priorities for effecting optimal ranges of information processing for organized function in the various units or structures making up the hierarchy of structures; they thereby give themselves the highest priority for experiencing optimal information-load.

In the human organism, the cerebral cortex would be the structure having highest priority for experiencing an optimal information load for organized function.

36

At one time in evolution, nocturnal enuresis may have performed a valuable function in that it aroused a deeply sleeping organism and thus allowed some scanning of the environment for potentially dangerous predators. Alternatively, a urine-soaked, sleeping organism might be less palatable to a predator than a dry or normal-smelling one. In modern times, nocturnal enuresis might be homeostatic only in its information processing function; enuresis is generally accompanied by increases in endogenous (awakenings) and exogenous (disturbed parents) sensory information flow.

37

The work of Charlotte Bach (cited in Wilson, 1978: 514-522) describes a theoretical framework which suggests that most so-called sexual perversions may be conceptualized as variations of normal sexual behavior.

38

Mathematical techniques such as topology, group, set and digraph theory, and classical calculus are used in system approaches. Multivariable problems require multivariate statistics and designs; computers and electronic simulation will necessarily play a large role in the development of this field. A comprehensive theory of systems does not exist today. Problems encountered (e.g., nonlinearity and large numbers appearing in system interactions) transcend presently available mathematics and require development.

39

Recently, Battista (1977) has proposed that structuralism may provide the foundation for a new and more encompassing form of general system theory, since it is able to represent the hierarchical evolution of systems. Structuralism, a method of analysis with historical roots in the Gestalt psychology of Kohler (and currently represented by Piaget's cognitive psychology, Chomsky's linguistics, and Levi-Strauss's anthropology) conceptualizes a system as a self-regulating set of transformations (Piaget, 1970). Battista (1977) suggests that Muses' (1968) hypernumber and metadimension theory in combination with Khinchin's (1957) approach to information promises the possibility of developing a formal representation of different hierarchical levels of structure, each associated with a different hierarchical level of information. Such an approach would be able to discuss the hierarchical development of a system as a function of the interaction of the environment with the system's information processing mechanisms.

40   Using strictly formal methods, Godel (1960) proved that any finite set of consistent axioms is incapable of implying all the true theorems of the theory of numbers. His theorem presents formal proof of a nonlogical component inherent in all logical systems, since he was able to show that there would be true statements about arithmetic, not deducible from that set of axioms.

41   It is not clear at this point whether all systems are incomplete. Godel's theorem applies to Western arithmetic systems.

42   Heisenberg demonstrated that the imprecision in one measurement multiplied by the imprecision in the other can never be less than Planck's Constant (h), a degree of uncertainty (h = 6.624×10^{-27} erg-second) considered to be negligible in all but atomic and subatomic instances.

43   Bell's theorem suggests that either the statistical predictions of quantum theory are false or the principle of "local causes" is false. The principle of local causes says that what happens in one area does not depend upon variables subject to the control of an experimenter in a distant space-like separated area.

44   One only has to look at ecological crises and the recent shortages of raw materials, oil and energy for confirmation of the systems approach premise of interdependence.

45   Petrinovich (1979) has recently critized the accepted research paradigm in behavioral science and pointed out its inherent limitations in light of findings in contemporary psychology and physics. An alternative paradigm is outlined and demonstrated to be adequate to the task of understanding organism-environment relationships. The alternative, formulated in terms of Brunwick's lens model, points out theoretical implications for future research method, including the importance of situational sampling, the nature and focus of analytical statistical procedures, and the characteristics of a molar functional approach as contrasted with those of a molecular reductionistic one.

46   Wachtel (1980) examines a number of prominent trends in the conduct of psychological research and considers how they may limit progress in the field of psychological science. He describes how failure to appreciate important differences in temperament and talent among researchers has prevented the development in psychology of a vigorous tradition of fruitful theoretical inquiry. Emphasis on quantitative "productivity"

or activity at the expense of thought, a problem for all disciplines, is shown to have had particularly unfortunate results in psychology, as has exclusive reliance on the experimental method for the generation of new ideas and the confirmation of old conceptualizations.

Bibliography

Abrams, R. D., Huebsch, R., & Raiken, B. L. Effect of electrical shock stress on transplanted tumors in mice. *Federation Proceedings,* 1961, *20,* 326.

Abse, D. W., Wilkins, M. M., Van De Castle, R. L., Buxton, W. D., Demars, J. P., Brown, R. S., & Kirschner, L. G. Personality and behavioral characteristics of lung cancer patients. *Journal of Psychosomatic Research,* 1974, *18,* 101-113.

Achterberg, J., Lawlis, G. F., Simon, O. C., & Simonton, S. Psychological factors and blood chemistries as disease outcome predictors for cancer patients. *Multivariate Clinical and Experimental Research,* 1977, *3,* 107-122.

Achterberg, J., & Lawlis, G. F. *Imagery of cancer (image-ca): an evaluation tool for the process of disease.* Champaign, Illinois: Institute for Personality and Ability Testing, 1978.

Achterberg, J., Simonton, O. C. & Matthews-Simonton, S. *Stress, psychological factors, and cancer.* Fort Worth, Texas: New Medicine Press, 1976.

Achor, R. W. P., Hanson, N. O., & Gifford, R. W. Hypertension treated with Rauwolfia serpentina (whole root) and with reserpine. *Journal of the American Medical Association,* 1955, *159,* 841-845.

Achterberg, J., Collerrain, I., & Craig, P. A possible relationship between cancer, mental retardation and mental disorder. *Social Science and Medicine,* 1978, *12,* 135-139.

Ader, R. Early experience and adaptation to stress. In *Endocrines and the Central Nervous System,* Vol. 43, issued by the Association for Research in Nervous and Mental Disorders. Baltimore: Williams & Wilkins, 1966, 292-306.

Ader, R., & Friedman, S. B. Psychological factors and susceptibility to disease in animals. In *Symposium on Medical Aspects of Stress in the Military Climate.* Washington, D.C., Walter Reed Army Institute of Research, 1964, 457.

Ader, R., & Friedman, S. B. Differential early experiences and susceptibility to transplanted tumor in the rat. *Journal of Comparative and Physiological Psychology,* 1965b, *59,* 361-364.

Ader, R., & Friedman, S. B. Social factors affecting emotionality and resistance to disease in animals V. Early separation from the mother and response to a transplanted tumor in the rat. *Psychosomatic Medicine,* 1965a, *27,* 119-122.

Aimez, P. Psychophysiology of cancer. *Revue Medicale Psychosomatique,* 1972, *14,* 371-381.

Albert, Z. Effect of injuries of primary neoplastic focus on growth metastases of tumor. II. biopsy of Crocker's sarcoma in mice. *Patalogia Polska,* 1956, *7,* 1-9.

Albert, Z., Medras, K., & Gorska, I. Further studies on the effect of environment on the development of spontaneous mammary cancer and malignant mesenchymal tumors in mice. *Acta Medica Polona,* 1962, *3,* 131-136.

Alexander L. Effects of psychotropic drugs on conditioned responses in man. In *Neuropsychopharmacology,* Vol. 2, Proceedings of the second meeting of the Collegium Internationale Neuropsychopharmacologicum. Balse, July 1960. E. Rothlin (Ed.), Amsterdam: Elsevier, 1961, 93-123

Allison J. Cognitive structure and receptivity to low intensity stimulation. *Journal of Abnormal and Social Psychology,* 1963, *67,* 132-138.

Alsop, S., *Stay of execution: a sort of memoir.* Philadelphia: J. B. Lippencott Co., 1973.

Amkraut, A., & Solomon, G. F. Stress and murine sarcoma virus (Moloney)-induced tumors. *Cancer Research,* 1972, *32,* 1428-1433.

Anderson, D. E. Genetic study of breast cancer—identification of a high risk group. *Cancer,* 1974, *34,* 1090-1097.

Andervont, H. B. Influence of environment on mammary cancer in mice. *Journal of the National Cancer Institute,* 1944, *4,* 579-581.

Andervont, H. B. Spontaneous tumors in a subline of strain C3H mice. *Journal of the National Cancer Institute,* 1941, *1,* 737-744.

Armstrong, B., Stevens, N., & Doll, R. Retrospective study of the association between the use of Rauwolfia derivatives and breast cancer in English women. *Lancet,* 1974, *2,* 672-675.

Aserinsky, E. The maximal capacity for sleep: rapid eye movement density as an index of sleep satiety. *Biological Psychiatry,* 1969, *1,* 147-159.

Aserinsky, E., & Kleitman, N. Regularly occurring periods of eye motility and concomitant phenomena during sleep. *Science,* 1953, *118,* 273-274.

Ashby, W. R. *Introduction to cybernetics.* New York: Methuen, 1968.

Bacon, C. L., Renneker, R., & Cutler, M. A psychosomatic survey of cancer of the breast. *Psychosomatic Medicine,* 1952, *14,* 453-460.

Baekeland, F. Exercise deprivation: sleep and psychological reactions. *Archives of General Psychiatry,* 1970, *22,* 365-369.

Baekeland, F., & Lasky, R. Exercise and sleep patterns in college athletes. *Perceptual and Motor Skills,* 1966, *23,* 1203-1207.

Bahnson, C. B. & Bahnson, M. B. Role of the ego defences—denial and repression in the etiology of malignant neoplasm. *Annals of the New York Academy of Sciences,* 1965, *125,* 827-845.

Bahnson, M. B. & Bahnson, C. B. Ego defenses in cancer patients.

Annals of the New York Academy of Sciences, 1969, *164,* 546-577.

Bahnson, C. B. Basic epistemological considerations regarding psychosomatic processes and their application to current psychophysiological cancer research. *International Journal of Psychobiology,* 1970, *1,* 57-69.

Bahnson, C. B., & Bahnson, M. B. Denial and repression of primitive impulses and of disturbing emotions in patients with malignant neoplasms. In D. M. Kissen & L. L. LeShan (Eds.), *Psychosomatic aspects of neoplastic disease.* London: Pitman Medical Publishing Company, 1964, 42-62.

Baldwin, R. W., Barker, C. P., & Embleton, M. J. Immunology of carcinogen-induced and spontaneous rat tumors. In J. Dausset, J. Hamburger, & G. Mathe (Eds.), *Advance in Transplantation; Proceedings of the First International Congress of the Transplantation Society,* June 27-30, 1967. Munksgaard: Copenhagen, 1967, 503-505.

Ban, T., & Shinoda, H. Experimental studies on the relation between the hypothalamus and conditioned reflex. *Medical Journal of Osaka University,* 1956, *1,* 643-676.

Barness, L. A., Morrow, G., & Clark, G. R. Biochemical basis of mental retardation. In J. Mendels (Ed.), *Biological psychiatry.* New York: John Wiley & Sons, 1973, 471.

Barrett, J. T. *Immunology: an introduction to immunochemistry and immunobiology.* St. Louis: The C. V. Mosby Company, 1974, 21-47.

Bartlett, F. C. *Remembering: a study in experimental and social psychology.* Cambridge, England: Cambridge University Press, 1932.

Bateson, G. *Steps to an ecology of mind.* New York: Ballantine Books, 1972.

Bateson, G. *Mind and nature: a necessary unity.* New York: E. P. Dutton, 1979.

Battista, J. R. The science of consciousness. In K. S. Pope & J. L. Singer (Eds.), *The stream of consciousness.* New York: Plenum, 1978, 55-87.

Battista, J. R. The holistic paradigm and general system theory. *General Systems,* 1977, *22,* 65-71.

Bauer, K. H. *Das krebsproblem.* Berlin: Springer-Verlag, 1963.

Baumler, E. *Cancer—A review of international research.* London: Queen Anne Press, 1968.

Beatson, G. T. On the treatment of inoperable cases of carcinoma of the mammaries: suggestions for a new method of treatment with illustrative cases. *Lancet,* 1896, *2,* 104-107.

Beck, A. T. *Depression—causes and treatment.* Philadelphia: University of Pennsylvania Press, 1967.

Beitman, B. D., & Carlin, A. S. Night terrors treated with imipramine. *American Journal of Psychiatry,* 1979, *136,* 1087-1088.

Belisario, J. *Cancer of the skin.* London: Butterworth and Company, 1959.

Benjamin, J. D. Developmental biology and psychoanalysis. In N. S. Greenfield & W. C. Lewis (Eds.), *Psychoanalysis and current biological thought.* Madison: University of Wisconsin Press, 1965.

Bennette, G. Psychic and cellular aspects of isolation and identity impairment in cancer—a dialectic of alienation. *Annals of the New York Academy of Sciences, 1969, 164,* 352-364.

Berenblum, I. *Carcinogenesis as a biological problem.* Oxford: North-Holland Publishing Company, 1974.

Berger, R. J. Oculomotor control: A possible function of REM sleep. *Psychological Review,* 1969, *76,* 144-164.

Berger, R. J., & Oswald, I. Eye movements during active and passive dreams. *Science,* 1962, *137,* 601.

Berlucchi, G., Moruzzi, G., Salvi, G., & Strata, P. Pupil behavior and ocular movements during synchronized and desynchronized sleep. *Archives Italiennes de Biologie,* 1964, *102,* 230-244.

Berlucchi, G., & Strata, P. Ocular phenomena during synchronized and desynchronized sleep. In *Centre National de la Recherche Scientifique. Aspects anatomo-fonctionnels de la physiologie du sommeil, Lyon.* Paris: Centre National de la Recherche, 1965, 285.

Berlyne, D. E. *Conflict, arousal, and curiosity.* New York: McGraw-Hill, 1960.

Bernstein, S., & Kaufman, M.R. A psychological analysis of apparent depression following Rauwolfia therapy. *Journal of the Mount Sinai Hospital, 1960, 27,* 525-530.

von Bertalanffy, L. An outline of general system theory. *British Journal for Philosophy of Science,* 1950, *1,* 139-164.

von Bertalanffy, L. The mind-body problem—a new view. *Psychosomatic Medicine,* 1964, *26,* 29-45.

von Bertalanffy, L. Principles and theory of growth. In W. W. Nowinski (Ed.), *Fundamental aspects of normal and malignant growth.* New York: Elsevier Publishing Co., 1960, 137-253.

von Bertalanffy, L. *Robots, men and minds.* New York: George Braziller, 1969.

Bjelke, E. Dietary vitamin A and human lung cancer. *International Journal of Cancer,* 1975, *15,* 561-565.

Blum, H. F. *Carcinogenesis by ultraviolet light.* Princeton: Princeton University Press, 1959.

Blum, J. S., Crow, K. L., & Pribram, K. H. A behavioral analyses of organization of parietal-temporal-preoccipital cortex. *Journal of Comparative Neurology,* 1950, *93,* 53-100.

Blumberg, E. M., West, P. M., & Ellis, F. W. A. (Eds.) MMPI findings in human cancer. In *Basic reading on the MMPI in psychology and medicine.* Minneapolis: Minnesota University Press, 1956, 452-460.

Blumberg, E. M., West, P. M., & Ellis, F. W. A. Possible relationship between psychological factors and human cancer. *Psychosomatic Medicine,* 1954, *16,* 277-286.

Bohm, D. Wholeness and the implicate order. London: Routledge &

Kegan Paul, 1980.

Bollag, W. Vitamin A and vitamin A acid in the prophylaxis and therapy of epithelial tumors. *International Journal of Vitamin Research*, 1970, *40*, 299-313.

Bonnett, M. H., & Webb, W. B. Effect of two experimental sets on sleep structure. *Perceptual and Motor Skills*, 1976, *42*, 343-350.

Bonvallet, M., Dell, P., & Hiebel, G. Sinus carotidien et activite electrique cerebrale. *Comptes Rendus des Seances de la Societe de Biologie*, 1953, *147*, 1166-1169.

Booth, G. Krebs and tuberkulose im rorschachschen formdeuteversuch. *Zeitschrift fur Psychosomatische Medizin und Psychoanalyse*, 1964, *10*, 176-188.

Borkovec, T. D. Autonomic reactivity to sensory stimulation in psychopathic and normal juvenile delinquents. *Journal of Consulting and Clinical Psychology*, 1970, *35*, 217-222.

Brady, J. V. Psychophysiology of emotional behavior. In A. J. Bachrach (Ed.), *Experimental foundations of clinical psychology*. New York: Basic Books, 1962, 47-63.

Brady, J. V., Porter, R. W., Conrad, D. G., & Mason, J. W. Avoidance behavior and the development of gastroduodenal ulcers. *Journal of the Experimental Analysis of Behavior*, 1958, *1*, 69-72.

Brain W. R., Daniel, P. M., & Greenfield, J. B. Subacute cortical cerebellar degeneration and its relation to carcinoma. *Journal of Neurology, Neurosurgery and Psychiatry*, 1951, *14*, 59-75.

Broadbent, D. E. Information processing in the nervous system. *Science*, 1965, *150*, 457-462.

Broadbent, D. E. *Perception and communication*. Oxford: Pergamon Press, 1958.

Broughton, R. Confusional sleep disorders: interrelationship with memory consolidation and retrieval in sleep. In T. J. Boag & D. Campbell (Eds.), *A triune concept of the brain and behavior*. Toronto: University of Toronto Press, 1973.

Broughton, R. Biorhythmic variations in consciousness and psychological functions. *Canadian Psychological Review*, 1976, *16*, 217-239.

Broughton, R. J., Poire, R., & Tassinari, C. A. The electrodermogram (Tarchanoff effect) during sleep. *Electroencephalography and Clinical Neurophysiology*, 1965, *18*, 691-708.

Browman, C. P. Sleep following sustained exercise. *Psychophysiology*, 1980, *17*, 577-580.

Brown, B. *Supermind: the ultimate energy*. New York: Harper & Row, 1980.

Brown, F. The relationship between cancer and personality. *Annals of the New York Academy of Sciences*, 1965, *125*, 865-873.

Buinauskas, P., McDonald, G. O., & Cole, W. H. Role of operative stress on the resistance of the experimental animal to inoculated cancer cells. *Annals of Surgery*, 1958, *148*, 642-645.

Burkitt, D. P. Epidemiology of cancer of the colon and rectum. *Cancer*, 1971, *28*, 3-13.

Burnet, F. M. A modern basis for pathology. *Lancet,* 1968, *1,* 1383-1387.

Buss, A. H. *Psychopathology.* New York: John Wiley & Sons, 1966, 345.

Butler, S., *Evolution, old and new.* New York: E. P. Dutton & Co., 1924.

Cameron, E. *Hyaluronidase and cancer.* New York: Pergamon Press, 1966.

Cameron, E., & Rotman, D. Ascorbic acid, cell proliferation and cancer. *Lancet,* 1972, *1,* 542.

Cameron, E., & Pauling, L. *Cancer and vitamin C.* Menlo Park, California: Linus Pauling Institute of Science and Medicine, 1979.

Campbell, J. A., & Cramer, W. Some effects of alteration of oxygen pressure in the inspired air upon cancer growth and body-weight of rats and mice. *Lancet,* 1928, *1,* 828-830.

Cancer Facts and Figures. *American Cancer Society, Inc.,* 1975, 22.

Capra, F. The new physics as a model for the new medicine. *Journal of Social and Biological Structures,* 1977, *1,* 1-8.

Capra, F. *The tao of physics.* Boulder, Colorado: Shambhela Publications, 1975.

Cardon, P. V., & Mueller, P. S. A possible mechanism—psychogenic fat mobilization. *Annals of the New York Academy of Sciences,* 1965, *125,* 924-927.

Charatan, F. B., & Brierley, J.B. Mental disorder associated with primary lung carcinoma. *British Medical Journal,* 1956, *1,* 765-768.

Chardin, T. *The phenomenon of man.* New York: Harper & Row, 1950.

Cherry, C. *On human communication.* Cambridge: Technology Press of Massachusetts Institute of Technology, 1957.

Chouroulinkov, I., Guillon, J. C., & Guerin, M. Endometrial sarcomas in mice—A survey of 130 cases. *Journal of the National Cancer Institute,* 1969, *42,* 593-603.

Christopherson, W. M., & Parker, J. E. Relation of cervical cancer to early marriage and childbearing. *New England Journal of Medicine,* 1965, *273,* 235-239.

Christopherson, W., & Mendez, W. A local geographic study of cervical cancer. *Bulletin of the International Academy of Pathology,* 1966, *7,* 103-105.

Wu C. Biochemical correlation of oncogenesis with ontogenesis. *International Journal of Cancer,* 1973, *11,* 438-447.

Claridge, G. B., & Hume, W. I. Comparison of effects of dexamphetamine and LSD-25 on perceptual and autonomic function. *Perceptual and Motor Skills,* 1966, *23,* 456-458.

Clayson, D. B. *Chemical carcinogenesis.* Boston: Little, Brown & Co., 1962.

Clelland, C. C., Powell, H. C., & Talhington, L. W. Death of the profoundly retarded. *Mental Retardation,* 1971, *9 (5),* 36.

Clemens, T. L. A preliminary report on autonomic functions in neoplastic diseases. In J. A. Gengerelli & F. J. Kirkner (Eds.), *The psychological variables in human cancer.* Berkeley: The University of California Press, 1954, 95-124.

Clemmesen, J. *Statistical studies in malignant neoplasms.* Copenhagen: Munkesgaard, 1965.

Cobb, B. *A socio-psychological study of the cancer patient.* Doctoral dissertation, University of Texas, Austin, 1952.

Coble, P., Foster, F. G., & Kupfer, D. J. Electroencephalographic sleep diagnosis of primary depression. *Archives of General Psychiatry,* 1976, *33,* 1124-1127.

Cohen, N. J., & Douglas, V. I. Characteristics of the orienting response in hyperactive and normal children. *Psychophysiology,* 1972, *9,* 238-245.

Cohnheim, J. *Lectures on general pathology* (A handbook for practitioners and students. Tr. from the 2nd German ed. by Alexander B. McKee.) London: The New Syndenham Society, 1889-90.

Collins, L. G., & Stone, L. A. Pain sensitivity, age, and activity level in chronic schizophrenics and in normals. *British Journal of Psychiatry,* 1966, *112,* 33-35.

Cone, M. U., & Nettesheim, P. Effects of vitamin A on 3-methylcholanthrene induced squamous cell metaplasias and early tumors in the respiratory tract of rats. *Journal of the National Cancer Institute,* 1973, *50,* 1599-1606.

Consumer Reports. Diet and heart disease. 1981, *41,* 256-260.

Coppen, A., & Metcalfe, M. Cancer and extraversion. *British Medical Journal,* 1963, *2,* 18-19.

Corson, S. A. Neuroendocrine and behavioral response patterns to psychologic stress and the problem of the target issue in cerebrovisceral pathology. *Annals of the New York Academy of Sciences,* 1965, *125,* 890-918.

Coursey, R. D., Buchsbaum, M., & Frankel, B. L. Personality measures and evoked responses in chronic insomniacs. *Journal of Abnormal Psychology,* 1975, *84,* 239-249.

Cousins, N. *Anatomy of an illness as perceived by the patient: reflections on healing & regeneration.* New York: W. W. Norton and Co., 1979.

Cowdry, E. V. *Etiology and prevention of cancer in man.* New York: Appleton-Century-Crofts, 1968.

Cowie, A. T. Hormonal factors in mammary development and lactation. In B. A. Stoll (Ed.), *Mammary cancer and neuroendocrine therapy.* London: Butterworth & Co., 1974, 13.

Crick, F. *Of molecules and men.* Seattle: University of Washington Press, 1966.

Crisp, A.H. Some psychosomatic aspects of neoplasia. *British Journal of Medical Psychology,* 1970, *43,* 313-331.

Cutler, M. The nature of cancer process in relation to a possible psychosomatic influence. In J. A. Gengerelli & F. J. Kirkner (Eds.), *Psychological variables in human cancer.* Berkeley and Los

Angeles: University of California Press, 1954, 1-16.

Czikszentmihalyi, M. Attention and the holistic approach to behavior. In K. S. Pope & J. L. Singer (Eds.), *The stream of consciousness.* New York: Plenum, 1978, 335-358.

Czikszentmihalyi, M. *Beyond boredom and anxiety: the experience of play in work and games.* San Francisco: Jossey-Bass, 1975.

Davidson, R. J., & Schwartz, G. E. The psychobiology of relaxation and related states. In D. Mostofsky (Ed.), *Behavior control and modification of physiological activity.*   Englewood, N.J.: Prentice-Hall, 1976.

Davies, R. K., Quinlan, D. M., McKegney, F. P., & Kimball, C. P. Organic factors and psychological adjustment in advanced cancer patients. *Psychosomatic Medicine,* 1973, *35*, 464-471.

Davis, C. L., & Bauman, D. E. General metabolism associated with the synthesis of milk. In B. L. Larson & V. R. Smith (Eds.), *Lactation—a comprehensive treatise* (Vol. 2). New York: Academic Press, 1974, 3-30.

Dawe, C. J. Invertebrate animals in cancer research. *Experimental Animal Cancer Research, Monograph,* 1968, *5*, 45-55.

Dawe, C. J. Phylogeny and oncogeny—in neoplasms and related disorders of invertebrate and lower vertebrate animals. *National Cancer Institute Monograph,* 1969, *31*, 1-40.

Dawson, G. D. The effect of cortical stimulation on transmission through the cuneate nucleus in the anesthetized rat. *Journal of Physiology,* 1958, *142*, 2-3.

Dawson, M. E., Schell, A. M., & Catemia, J. J.   Autonomic correlates of depression and clinical improvement following electroconvulsive shock therapy. *Psyschophysiology,* 1977, *14*, 569-578.

DeChambre, R. P., & Gosse, C. Individual versus group caging of mice with grafted tumors. *Cancer Research,* 1973, *33*, 140-144.

Deelman, H. T. The part played by injury and repair in the development of cancer. *British Medical Journal,* 1927, *1*, 872.

de la Peña, A., Zarcone, V., & Dement, W. C. Correlation between measures of the rapid eye movements of wakefulness and sleep. *Psychophysiology,* 1973, *10*, 488-500.

de la Peña, A. *The psycho-biological role of the rapid eye movement dream state.* Unpublished doctoral dissertation, Stanford University, 1971.

de la Peña, A., Flickinger, R., & Mayfield, D. Reverse first night effect in chronic poor sleepers. *Sleep Research,* 1977, *6*, 167.

de la Peña, A. & Ornitz, E. M. Effect of sensory enrichment and deprivation on REM sleep in autistic and normal children. Paper read at the Association for the Psychophysiological Study of Sleep meeting, San Diego, 1973.

de la Peña, A. Cholinergic dominance in the etiology of narcolepsy. *Sleep Research,* 1977, *6*, 166.

de la Peña, A. Varieties of aggressive men. *Contemporary Psychology,* 1979a, *24*, 660-661.

de la Peña, A. Unpublished data, 1980.

de la Peña, A. Unpublished data, 1979b.

de la Peña, A. Toward a psychophysiologic conceptualization of insomnia. In R. L. Williams & I. Karacan (Eds.), *Sleep disorders: diagnosis and treatment.* New York: John Wiley & Sons, 1978, 101-143.

Della Porta, G., & Terracini, B. Chemical carcinogenesis in infant animals. *Progress in Experimental Tumor Research,* 1969, *11,* 334-363.

Della Porta, G., Colnaghi, M. I., & Parmi, L. Influenza della timectomia, della splenectomia e del cortisone sulla cancerogenesi. *Tumori,* 1970, *56,* 121-135.

Dement, W. C. *Program notes: Elaboration of possible sleep mechanisms.* Paper presented to the 1969 American Medical Association Convention, New Brunswick, New Jersey, 1969.

Dement, W., Ferguson, J., Cohen, H., & Barchas, J. Non-chemical methods and data using a biochemical model: the REM quanta. In A. J. Mandell & M. P. Mandell (Eds.), *Psychochemical research in man: methods, strategy, and theory.* New York: Academic Press, 1969, 275-325.

Depue, R. A., & Fowles, D. C. Conceptual ability, response interference, and arousal in withdrawn and active schizophrenics. *Journal of Consulting and Clinical Psychology,* 1974, *42,* 509-518.

Dewan, E. Consciousness as an emergent causal agent in the context of control system theory. In G. Globus (Ed.), *Brain and conscious experience.* New York: Plenum Press, 1976.

Dewson, J. H., III, Nobel, K. W., & Pribram, K. H. Corticofugal influence at cochlear nucleus of the cat—some effects of ablation of insular-temporal cortex. *Brain Research,* 1966, *2,* 151-159.

Doderlein, G. Lerr kreus der weissen mousetsch. *Zeitschrift fur Krebsforschung,* 1926, *23,* 241.

Doll, R., & Hill, A. B. (Cited in Fisher, R. A.). *Smoking—The cancer controversy.* Edinburgh: Oliver and Boyd, 1959.

Doll, R. The geographical distribution of cancer. *British Journal of Cancer,* 1969, *23,* 1-8.

Donati, M. B., Davidson, J. F., & Garattini, S. (Eds.), *Malignancy and the hemostatic system.* New York: Raven Press, 1981.

Dorus, E., Dorus, W., & Rechtschaffen, A. The incidence of novelty in dreams. *Archives of General Psychiatry,* 1971, *25,* 364-368.

Dowben, R. M. *Cell biology.* New York: Harper & Row, 1971, 455.

Dragstedt, L. R. A concept of the etiology of gastric and duodenal ulcer. *American Journal of Roentgenology,* 1956, *75,* 219-229.

Dubrenilk, W. Epitheliomatore d'origine solaire. *Annales de Dermatologie et de Syphiligraphie* (8 Series), 1907, *4,* 387-391.

Dudley, D. L., Holmes, T. H., Martin, C. J., & Ripley, H.S. Changes in respiration associated with hypnotically induced emotion, pain, and exercise. *Psychosomatic Medicine,* 1964, *26,* 46-57.

Duffy, E. *Activation and behavior.* New York: John Wiley & Sons, 1962, 119-136.

Dunham, L. J., & Stewart, H. L.   A survey of transplantable and transmissible animal tumors.   *Journal of the National Cancer Institute,* 1953, *13,* 1299-1377.

Dworkin, B. R., Filewich, R. J., Miller, N. E., Craigmyle, N., & Pickering, T. G.   Baroreceptor activation reduces reactivity to noxious stimulation: implication for hypertension.   *Science,* 1979, *205,* 1299-2301.

Ebbesen, P., & Rask-Nielsen, R.   Influence of sex-segregated grouping and of inoculation with subcellular leukemic material on development of nonleukemic lesions in DBA/2, BALB/C, and CBA mice.   *Journal of the National Cancer Institute,* 1967, *39,* 917-932.

Eckman, P., & Hoppe, E.   Decreased resistance to inoculated Walker 256 carcinosarcoma cells subjected to traumatic stress.   *Proceedings of the American Association for Cancer Research,* 1959, *3,* 222.

Eichorn, D. H.   Berkeley longitudinal studies—continuities and correlates of behavior.   *Canadian Journal of Behavioral Science,* 1973, *5,* 297-320.

Eisdorfer, C.   The WAIS performance of the aged: A retest evaluation.   *Journal of Gerontology,* 1963, *18,* 169-172.

Elliot, J. A., & Welton, D. G.   Epithelioma—report on 1,742 treated patients.   *Archives of Dermatology and Syphilology,* 1946, *53,* 307-332.

Elsasser, W. M.   *The physical foundation of biology.*   New York: Pergamon Press, 1958.

Engle, G. L.   The need for a new medical model: a challenge for biomedicine.   *Science,* 1977, *196,* 129-136.

Engle, G. L.   A unified concept of health and disease.   *Perspectives in Biology and Medicine,* 1969, *3,* 459-485.

Epstein, S.   (Braslau) Die bezrehungen von haar—und hautfarbe zum hautepitheliom.   *Archiv fur Dermatologie und Syphilis,* 1931, *164,* 304-309.

Everett, H.   Relative state formulation of quantum mechanics.   *Review of Modern Physics,* 1957, *29,* 424-462.

Ewing, J.   *Neoplastic diseases* (4th ed., Chapters 1, 6, 7, and 8).   Philadelphia and London: W. B. Saunders, 1940.

Eysenck, H. J.   *The biological basis of personality.*   Springfield, Ill.: Charles C. Thomas, 1967.

Eysench, H. J.   *The manual of the Maudsley personality inventory.*   London: University of London Press, 1959.

Eysenck, S. B. G.   The validity of a personality questionnaire as determined by the method of nominated groups.   *Life Sciences,* 1962, *1,* 13-18.

Fabrega, H.   The need for an ethnomedical science.   *Science,* 1972, *189,* 169.

Fabrega, H.   The portion of psychiatry in the understanding of human disease.   *Archives of General Psychiatry,* 1975, *35,* 1500.

Fadeeva, V. N.   *Pavlov Journal of Higher Nervous Activity,* 1951, *1,*

165.

Farley, F., & Farley, S. V.   Extroversion and stimulus-seeking motivation. *Journal of Consulting Psychology,* 1967, *31,* 215-216.

Farquhar, J. U., Wood, P. D., Breitose, H., et al.   Community education for cardiovascular health. *Lancet,* 1977, *2,* 1192-1195.

Feinberg, I., & Carlson, V. R.   Sleep variables as a function of age in man. *Archives of General Psychiatry,* 1969, *18,* 239-250.

Fernstrom, J. D., & Wurtman, R. J.   Brain serotonin content: physiological regulation by plasma neutral amino acids. *Science,* 1972, *178,* 414-416.

Fernstrom, J. D., & Wurtman, R. J.   Nutrition and the brain. *Scientific American,* 1974, *230,* 84-91.

Fessel, W. J.   Mental stress, blood proteins, and the hypothalamus. *Archives of General Psychiatry,* 1962, *7,* 427-435.

Fessel, W. J., & Forsyth, R. P.   Hypothalamic role in control of gamma globulin levels. *Arthritis and Rheumatism,* 1963, *6,* 771-772.

Fibiger, H. C., Lytle L. D., & Campbell, B. A.   Cholinergic modulation of adrenergic arousal in the developing rat. *Journal of Comparative and Physiological Psychology,* 1970, *72,* 384-389.

Finch, S. M.   Psychophysiologic disorders in children and adolescents. In Z. J. Lipowski (Ed.), *Psychosomatic medicine: current trends and clinical applications.* New York: Oxford University Press, 1977, 497-509.

Finkel, M. P., & Scribner, G. M.   Mouse cages and spontaneous tumors. *British Journal of Cancer,* 1955, *9,* 464-472.

Finstad, J.   Further phylogenetic studies of susceptibility and resistance to total body irradiation. *Federation Proceedings,* 1969, *28,* 751.

Fischer, R., Marks, P. A., Hill, R. M., & Rockey, M. A.   Personality structure as the main determinant of drug-induced (model) psychoses. *Nature,* 1968, *218,* 296-298.

Fisher, B., & Fisher, E. R.   Experimental evidence in support of the dormant tumor cell. *Science,* 1959, *130,* 918-919.

Fisher, J. G., de la Peña, A., & Donovan, W. N.   The role of trauma in obesity associated with sleep apnea. *Sleep Research,* 1977, *6,* 168.

Fiske, D. W., & Maddi, S. R.   *Functions of varied experience.* Homewood, Illinois: Dorsey Press, 1961.

Fleming, I. D., Barnawell, J. R., Burlison, P. E., & Rankin, J. S.   Skin cancer in black patients. *Cancer,* 1975, *35,* 600-605.

Forbes, T. R.   Physiology of reproduction in the female. In T. C. Ruch & H. D. Patton (Eds.), *Physiology and biophysics,* (19th edition). Philadelphia: W. B. Saunders Co., 1966, 1199-1200.

Ford, A.   Attention-automatization: an investigation of the transitional nature of mind. *American Journal of Psychology,* 1929, *41,* 1-31.

Foster, F. G., Kupfer, D. J., Coble, P., & McPartland, R. J.   Rapid eye movement sleep density: an objective indicator in severe medical-depressive syndromes. *Archives of General Psychiatry,* 1976, *33,* 1119-1123.

Foulds, L. The experimental study of tumor progression—a review. *Cancer Research,* 1954, *14,* 327-339.

Foulkes, W. D. Dream reports from different stages of sleep. *Journal of Abnormal and Social Psychology,* 1962, *65,* 14-25.

Foulkes, W. D., & Pope, R. PVE and SCE in stage REM: a modest confirmation and an extension. *Sleep Research,* 1972, *1,* 103.

Fox, B. H. Premorbid psychological factors as related to incidence of cancer. *Journal of Behavioral Medicine,* 1978, *1,* 45-133.

Fraumeni, J. F., Lloyd, J. W., Smith, E. M., & Wagoner, J. K. Cancer mortality among nuns—Role of marital status in etiology of neoplastic disease in women. *Journal of the National Cancer Institute,* 1969, *42,* 455-468.

Frederickson, C. J., Madansky, D. L., & Rechtschaffen, A. Sensory stimulation and subsequent sleep. *Communications in Behavioral Biology,* 1969, *4,* 109-113.

Freeman, A. E., Price, P. J., Bryan, R. J., Gordon, R. J., Gilden, R. J., Kelloff, G. J., & Huebner, R. J. Transformation of rat and hamster embryo cells by extracts of city smog. *Proceedings of the National Academy of Sciences of the United States of America,* 1971, *68,* 445-449.

Freis, E. D. Mental depression in hypertensive patients treated for long periods with large doses of reserpine. *New England Journal of Medicine,* 1954, *251,* 1006-1008.

Freud, S. *Mourning and melancholia.* London: Hogarth Press and the Institute of Psychoanalysis, 1917.

Frith, C. D. Smoking behavior and its relation to the smoker's immediate experience. *British Journal of Social and Clinical Psychology,* 1971, *10,* 73-78.

Fulton, J. F., Jacobsen, C. F., & Kennard, M. A. A note concerning the relation of the frontal lobes to posture and forced grasping in monkeys. *Brain,* 1932, *55,* 524-536.

Funkenstein, D. H., Greenblatt, M., Solomon, H. C, Autonomic nervous system changes following electric shock treatment. *Journal of Nervous and Mental Disease,* 1948, *108,* 409-422.

Funkenstein, D. H., Greenblatt, M., Solomon, H.C. Psychophysiological study of mentally ill patients. I. The status of the peripheral autonomic nervous system as determined by the reaction to epinephrine and mecholyl. *American Journal of Psychiatry,* 1949, *106,* 16-28.

Furst, C. Automatizing of visual attention (Doctoral Dissertation, Stanford University, 1970). *Dissertation Abstracts International,* 1970, *31,* 2304-B. (University Microfilms No. 70-18, 407).

Furst, C. Automatizing of visual attention. *Perception and Psychophysics,* 171, *10,* 65-70.

Furst, C. *Origins of the mind: mind-brain connections.* Englewood Cliffs: Prentice-Hall, 1979.

Gaarder, K. R. *Eye movements, vision, and behavior: a hierarchical visual information processing model*. New York: Halstead Press, 1975, 1-16.

Gagnon, F. Contribution to the study of the etiology and prevention of cancer of the cervix of the uterus. *American Journal of Obstetrics and Gynecology*, 1950, *60*, 516-522.

Galambos, R. Suppression of auditory nerve activity by stimulation of efferent fibers to the cochlea. *Federation Proceedings*, 1955, *14*, 53.

Galambos, R. Suppression of auditory nerve activity by stimulation of efferent fibers to the cochlea. *Federation Proceedings*, 1955, *14*, 53.

Galin, D. Background and evoked activity in the auditory pathway— Effects of noise shock-pairing. *Science*, 1965, *149*, 761-763.

Gardner, W. U. Hormonal aspects of experimental tumorigenesis. *Advances in Cancer Research*, 1953, *1*, 173-232.

Gastaut, H., & Bert, J. Electroencephalographic detection of sleep induced by repetitive sensory stimuli. In G. E. W. Wolstenholme & M. O'Connor (Eds.), *The nature of sleep*. Boston: Little, Brown & Co., 1960.

Gatlin, L. L. *Information theory and the living system*. New York: Columbia University Press, 1972, 25-49.

Gellhorn, E. *Autonomic regulations: their significance for physiology, psychology and neuropsychiatry*. New York: Interscience Publishers, 1943.

Gellhorn, E., & Kiely, W. Autonomic nervous system in psychiatric disorder. In J. Mendels (Ed.), *Biological psychiatry*. New York: John Wiley & Sons, 1973, 235-261.

Gellhorn, E., & Loofbourrow, G. N. *Emotions and emotional disorders*. New York: Harper & Row, 1963.

Gellhorn, E., Nakao, E., & Redgate, E. The influence of lesions in the anterior and posterior hypothalamus on tonic and phasic autonomic reactions. *Journal of Physiology*, 1956, *131*, 402-423.

Gellin, G., Kopf, A., & Garfinkel, L. Basal cell epithelioma—a controlled study of associated factors. In W. Montagna & R. Dobson (Eds.), *Advances in Biology of Skin* (Vol. 7). New York: Pergamon Press, 1966, 329-344.

Gengerelli, J. A., & Kirkner, F. J. *The psychological variables in human cancer*. Berkeley: The University of California Press, 1954.

Genzmer, A. *Untersuchrengen uber die sinneswahrnehmungen des neugebarenen menschen* (Dissertation, 1873). Halle: Niemeyer, 1882.

George, R. W. Cancer and other disorders related to certain perceptual tests. *Perceptual and Motor Skills*, 1970, *30*, 155-161.

Gerson, M. *Cancer therapy, results of fifty cases*. Del Mar, California: Totality Books, 1958.

Gilbert, D. G., Paradoxical tranquilizing and emotion-reducing effects of nicotine. *Psychological Bulletin*, 1979, *86*, 643-661.

Glemser, B. (Ed.) *Man against cancer*. New York: Funk and

Wagnalls, 1969, 311-312.

Globus, G. G. Mind, structure and contradictions. In G. G. Globus, G. Maxwell, & I. Savodnik (Eds.), Consciousness and the brain. New York: Plenum, 1976, 271-294.

Globus, G. Consciousness and brain. Archives of General Psychiatry, 1973, 29, 153-160.

Globus, G. The problem of consciousness. Psychoanalysis and contemporary science, 1974, 3, 40-69.

Godel, K. On formally undecidable propositions. New York: Basic Books, 1962.

Goffman, J. W., & Tamplin, A. R. Low dose radiation and cancer. New York Institute for Electrical and Electronic Engineers, Transactions on Nuclear Science, 1970a, NS17 (1), 1.

Goffman, J. W., & Tamplin, A. R. Federal radiation council guidelines for radiation exposure of the population—at large—protection or disaster? (Underground Uses of Nuclear Energy, Part 1). Washington, D.C., U.S. Government Printing Office, 1970b, 58-73.

Goldhaber, P. The influence of pore size on carcinogenicity of subcutaneously implanted millipore filters. Proceedings of the American Association for Cancer Research, 1959, 3, 228.

Goldin, A., Burton, R. M., Humphrey, S. R., & Venditti, J. M. Antileukemic action of reserpine. Science, 1957, 125, 156-157.

Good, R. A., & Finstad, J. Essential relationship between the lymphoid system, immunity, and malignancy. National Cancer Institute Monograph, 1969, 31, 41-58.

Gordon, A. S. Some aspects of hormonal influences upon the leukocytes. Annals of the New York Academy of Sciences, 1955, 59, 907-927.

Gottfried, B., & Molomut, N. Effects of surgical trauma and other environmental stressors on tumor growth and wound healing. Acta Unio Internationalis Contra Cancrum, 1964, 20, 1617-1620.

Gralnick, H. R. Cancer cell procoagulant activity. In Donati, M. B., Davidson, T. F., & Garattini, S. (Eds.), Malignancy and the hemostatic system. New York: Raven Press, 1981.

Granit, R., & Phillips, C. G. Excitatory and inhibitory processes acting upon individual Purkinje cells of the cerebellum in cats. Journal of Physiology, 1956, 133, 520-547.

Gray, J. A. Strength of the nervous system, introversion-extraversion, conditionability and arousal. Behaviour Research and Therapy, 1967, 5, 151-169.

Greene, W. A., & Miller, G. Psychological factors and reticuloendothelial disease. IV. Observations on a group of children and adolescents with leukemia. An interpretation of disease development in terms of the mother-child unit. Psychosomatic Medicine, 1958, 20, 124-144.

Greene, W. A. The psychosocial setting of the development of leukemia and lymphoma. Annals of the New York Academy of Sciences, 1965, 125, 794-801.

Greer, S., & Morris, T. Psychological attributes of women who develop breast cancer: a controlled study. *Journal of Psychosomatic Research*, 1975, *19*, 147-153.

Gruzelier, J. H., & Venables, P. H. Evidence of high and low levels of physiological arousal in schizophrenics. *Psychophysiology*, 1975, *12*, 66-73.

Hafner, H. Psychopathologie des stirnhirms 1939 bis 1955. Fortshritte der Neurologie und Psychiatrie ihrer Grenzgebiete, 1957, *25*, 205-252.

Hagnell, O. The premorbid personality of persons who develop cancer in a total population investigated in 1947 and 1957. *Annals of the New York Academy of Sciences*, 1965, *125*, 846-855.

Hall, A. F. Relationships of sunlight, complexion, and heredity to skin carcinogenesis. *Archives of Dermatology and Syphilology*, 1950, *61*, 589-610.

Hamilton, J. A. Attention, personality and the self-regulation of mood: absorbing interest and boredom. In Mather, B. A. (Ed.), *Progress in experimental personality research*. New York: Academic Press, 1981, *10*, 281-315.

Hammond, E. C. Smoking in relation to the death rates of one million men and women. In W. Haenszel (Ed.), *Epidemiological approaches to the study of cancer and other diseases*. (National Cancer Institute Monograph 19). Bethesda, Maryland: National Cancer Institute, 1966, 127-204.

Hanna, T. (Ed.) *Bodies in revolt*. New York: Dell Publishing Co., 1970.

Haran-Ghera, N., & Lurie, M. Effect of heterologous antithymocyte serum on mouse skin tumorigenesis. *Journal of the National Cancer Institute*, 1971, *46*, 103-112.

Hare, R. D. Psychopathy. In P. H. Venables & M. J. Christie (Eds.), *Research in Psychophysiology*. New York: John Wiley & Sons, 1975, 325-342.

Harkonen, P., & Konttinen, Y. The effect of lysergic acid diethylamide on the white blood cell count of the guinea pig. *Acta Pharmacologica et Toxicologica*, 1957, *14*, 104-111.

Harman, W. The new Copernican revolution. In C. Muses & A. M. Young (Eds.), *Consciousness and reality*. New York: Discus, 1974.

Harrington, R. L., Koreneff, C., Nasser, S., Wright, C., & Engelhard, C. *Project M824109: Systems Approach to Mental Health Care in an HMO Model*. Washington, D.C., NIMH, March, 1977.

Harris, S. Personal communication, June 1978.

Hartley, R. V. Transmission of information. *Bell Systems Technology Journal*, 1928, *5*, 126-133.

Hartmann, H. *Ego psychology and the problem of adaptation*. New York: International Universities Press, 1958. Translation of original 1939 publication.

Harvey, H., & Field, M. *The effects of stress on tumor development—data and methodological implications*. Paper delivered at the Western Psychological Association Meeting, 1957.

Harvey, O. J., Hunt, D. E., & Schroder, H. M. *Conceptual systems and personality organization.* New York: John Wiley & Sons, 1961.

Haslam, D. Age and the perception of pain. *Psychonomic Science,* 1969, *15,* 86-87.

Haslam, D. R. Individual differences in pain threshold and level of arousal. *British Journal of Psychology,* 1967, *58,* 139-142.

Hatch, A., Wiberg, G. S., Balazs, T., & Grice, H. C. Long term isolation stress in rats. *Science,* 1963, *142,* 507.

Hauri, P. The influence of evening activity on the onset of sleep. *Psychophysiology,* 1969, *5,* 426-430.

Hauri, P. Sleep in depression. *Psychiatric Annals,* 1974, *4,* 45-62.

Hauri, P., & Hawkins, D. R. Phasic REM, depression, and the relationship between sleeping and waking. *Archives of General Psychiatry,* 1971, *25,* 56-63.

Hauri, P., & Olmstead, E. The reverse first night effect in insomnia. Paper read at APSS Annual Meeting, Hyannis, Massachusetts, June, 1981.

Hawkins, D. R., & Mendels, J. Sleep disturbance in depressive syndromes. *The American Journal of Psychiatry,* 1966, *123,* 682-690.

Hawkins, D. R., Mendels, J., Scott, J., Bensch, G., & Teachey, W. The psychophysiology of sleep in psychotic depression: a longitudinal study. *Psychosomatic Medicine,* 1967, *29,* 329-344.

Heath, R. G. Development toward new physiologic treatments in psychiatry. *Journal of Neuropsychiatry,* 1964a, *5,* 318-331.

Heath, R. G. Factors altering brain function and behavior in schizophrenia. In P. Solomon & B. Glueck (Eds.), *Recent research on schizophrenia.* Psychiatric Research Report Number 19. Washington, D.C.: The American Psychiatric Association, 1964b, 178-179.

Hebb, D. O. Drives and the CNS (conceptual nervous system). *Psychological Review,* 1955, *62,* 243-254.

Hebb, D. O., & Thompson, W. R. The social significance of animal studies. In G. Lindzey & E. Aaronson (Eds.), *Handbook of social psychology.* Reading, Massachusetts: Addison-Wesley, 1954, 551-562.

Heidelberger, C., & Moldenhauer, M. G. The interaction of carcinogenic hydrocarbons with tissue constituents—IV—A quantitative study of the binding to skin proteins of several C14-labeled hydrocarbons. *Cancer Research,* 1956, *16,* 442-449.

Heinonen, O., Shapiro, S., Tuominen, L., & Turunen, M. Reserpine use in relation to breast cancer. *Lancet,* 1974, *2,* 675-677.

Heisenberg, W. *Across the frontier.* New York: Harper & Row, Tr. by Peter Health, 1975, 68.

Heisenberg, W. *Physics and philosophy.* New York: Harper & Row, 1958.

Hellman, L. M., Rosenthal, A. H., Kistner, R. W., & Gordon, R. Some factors influencing the proliferation of the reserve cells in the human cervix. *American Journal of Obstetrics and Gynecology,* 1954, *67,* 899-915.

Hemphill, R. E., Hall, K. R. L., & Crookes, T. G.   A preliminary report on fatigue and pain tolerance in depressive and psychoneurotic patients. *Journal of Mental Science,* 1952, *98,* 433-440.

Henry, J. P., Stephens, P. M., & Watson, F. M. C.   Force breeding, social disorder and mammary tumor formation in CBA/USC mouse colonies: a pilot study. *Psychosomatic Medicine,* 1975, *37,* 277-283.

Hernandez-Peon, R.   Psychiatric implication of neuropsychological research. *Bulletin of the Menninger Clinic,* 1964, *28,* 165-185.

Hilgard, E. R.   Consciousness in contemporary psychology. *Annual Review of Psychology,* 1980, *31,* 1-26.

Hinchcliffe, R.   The pattern of the threshold of perception for hearing and other special senses as a function of age. *Gerontologia,* 1958, *2,* 311-320.

Hinton, J. M.   *Dying.* (Rev. ed.). New York, Penguin Books, 1967.

Hinton, J. M.   The physical and mental distress of the dying. *Quarterly Journal of Medicine,* 1963, *32,* 1-21.

Hoffer, A.   The psychophysiology of cancer. *Journal of Asthma Research,* 1971, *8,* 61-76.

Hoffman, D., & Wynder, E. L.   Chemical analysis and carcinogenic bioassays of organic particulate pollutants. In A. C. Stern (Ed.), *Air pollution.* New York and London: Academic Press, 1968, (Vol. 2), 187-247.

Hoffman, S. A., Raschkis, K. E., De Bias, D. A., Cantarow, A., & Williams, T. L.   The influence of exercise on the growth of transplanted rat tumors. *Cancer Research,* 1962, *22,* 597-599.

Holcomb (Hamilton), J. A.   Attention and intrinsic rewards in the control of psychophysiologic states. *Psychotherapy and Psychosomatics,* 1977, *27,* 54-61.

Horne, J. A., & Porter, J. M.   Exercise and human sleep. *Nature,* 1975, *256,* 573-575.

Horne, J. A., & Walmsley, B.   Daytime visual load and the effects upon human sleep. *Psychophysiology,* 1976, *13,* 115-120.

Huebner, R. J., Freeman, A. E., Whitmire, C. E., Price, P. J., Khim, J. S., Kelloff, G. J., Gilden, R. V., & Meier, H.   In *Environment and cancer,* a symposium on fundamental cancer research sponsored by the University of Texas, M.D.   Anderson Hospital and Tumor Institute, Houston, Texas. Baltimore: Williams & Wilkins Company, 1972, 318-345.

Huggins, C. B.   Propositions in hormonal treatment of advanced cancers. *Journal of the American Medical Association,* 1965, *192,* 1141-1145.

Ikard, F. F., Green, D. E., & Horn, D.   A scale to differentiate between types of smoking as related to the management of affect. *International Journal of the Addictions,* 1969, *4,* 649-659.

Ikard, F. F., & Thompkins, S.   The experience of affect as a determinant of smoking behavior: a series of validity studies.

Journal of Abnormal Psychology, 1973, *81,* 172-181.

Illich, I.   *Medical nemesis: the expropriation of health.* New York: Pantheon Books, 1976.

Ingelfinger, F. J.   Health: a matter of statistics or feeling.   *New England Journal of Medicine,* 1977, *296,* 448-449.

Ivanov-Smolensky, A.   *Essays on the pathophysiology of the higher nervous activity.*   Moscow, Foreign Languages Publishing House, 1954.

Jacob, F., & Monod, J.   On the regulation of gene activity.   Cold Spring Harbor Symposium.   *Quantitative Biology,* 1961, *26,* 193-211.

James, W.   *Principles of psychology.*   New York: Holt, Rinehart & Winston, 1980.

Jantsch, Erich.   The self-organizing universe: scientific and human implications of the emerging paradigm of evolution.   Oxford, England: Pergamon Press, 1980.

Jarvie, H. F.   Frontal lobe wounds causing disinhibition.   *Journal of Neurology, Neurosurgery, and Psychiatry,* 1954, *17,* 14-32.

Jarvik, L. F., & Falek, A.   Cited in Baumler, E.   *Cancer—a review of international research.*   London: Queen Anne Press, 1968, 98-99.

Jensen, K.   Depressions in patients treated with reserpine for arterial hypertension.   *Acta Psychiatrica et Neurologica Scandinavica,* 1959, *34,* 195-204.

Jick, H., Slone, P., Shapiro, S., & Heinonen, O.   Reserpine and breast cancer.   *Lancet,* 1974, *2,* 669-672.

John, R.   A model of consciousness.   In G. Schwartz and D. Shapiro (Eds.), *Consciousness and self-regulation.*   New York: Plenum, 1976.

Johnson, L. C.   Are stages of sleep related to waking behavior?   *American Scientist,* 1973, *61,* 326-338.

Jones, A.   Stimulus-seeking behavior.   In J. P. Zubek (Ed.), *Sensory deprivation—fifteen years of research.* New York: Appleton-Century-Croft, 1969, 167-206.

Jones, A., & McGill, D. W.   The homeostatic character of information drive in humans.   *Journal of Experimental Research in Personality,* 1967, *2,* 25-31.

Jones, A., Wilkinson, H. J., & Braden, I.   Information deprivation as a motivational variable.   *Journal of Experimental Psychology,* 1961, *62,* 126-137.

Jones, A.   Stimulus-seeking behavior.   In J. P. Zubek, *Sensory deprivation—fifteen years of research.*   New York: Appleton-Century-Croft, 1969, 167-206.

Jones, B. M., Parsons, O. A., & Rundell, O. H.   Psychophysiological correlates of alcoholism.   In R. E. Tarter and A. A. Sugarman (Eds.), *Alcoholism: interdisciplinary approaches to an enduring problem.*   Reading, Massachusetts: Addison-Wesley, 1976, 435-477.

Jones, C. H.   The Funkenstein test in selecting methods of psychiatric treatment.   *Diseases of the Nervous System* 1956, *17,* 37-43.

Josephy, H. Analysis of mortality and causes of death in a mental hospital. *American Journal of Psychiatry*, 1949, *106*, 185-189.

Jung, R., & Baumgartner, G. Hemmungsmechanismen und bremsende stabilisierung an einzelnen neuronen des optischen cortex. *Pfluegers Archiv*, 1955, *261*, 434-456.

Jurko, M., Jost, H., & Hill, T. S. Pathology of the energy system—an experimental study of physiological adaptive capacities in a non-patient, a psycho-neurotic, and an early paranoid schizophrenic group. *The Journal of Psychology*, 1952, *33*, 183-198.

Kacser, H. Some physio-chemical aspects of biological organization. In C. H. Waddington (Ed.), *The strategy of the genes.* Great Britain: J. W. Arrowsmith, 1957, 224-235.

Kaliss, N., & Fuller, J. L. Incidence of lymphatic leukemia and methylcholanthrene-induced cancer in laboratory mice subjected to stress. *Journal of the National Cancer Institute*, 1968, *41*, 967-983.

Kaliss, N. Immunologic enhancement and inhibition of tumor growth—relationship to various immunological mechanisms. *Federation Proceedings*, 1965, *24*, 1024-1029.

Kaplan, H. S. On the natural history of the murine leukemia. Presidential Address. *Cancer Research*, 1967, *27*, 1325-1340.

Kaplan, H. S. Some possible mechanisms of carcinogenesis. In P. Emmelot & O. Muhlbock (Eds.), *Cellular control mechanisms and cancer.* New York: Elsevier, 1964, 373-382.

Kaplan, H. S., Nagareda, C. S., & Brown, M. B. The role of hormones in blood and blood-forming organs—endocrine factors and radiation-induced lymphoid tumors of mice. *Recent Progress in Hormone Research*, 1954, *10*, 293-338.

Kaliss, N. K. Immunologic enhancement and inhibition of tumor growth—relationship to various immunologic mechanisms. *Federation Proceedings*, 1965, *24*, 1024-1029.

Kaswan, J., Haralson, S., & Cline, R. Variables in perceptual and cognitive organization and differentiation. *Journal of Personality*, 1965, *33*, 164-177.

Kavetskii, R. E. Some problems of tumor pathogenesis. In R. E. Kavetskii (Ed.), *Neoplastic process and the nervous system.* Washington, D.C.: Washington Natural Science Foundation, 1960, 2-11.

Kavetskii, R. E. (Ed.). *The neoplastic process and the nervous system.* Kiev, USSR: State Medical Publishing House, 1958.

Kavetskii, R. E. *Tumors and the nervous system.* Kiev, USSR: Gos Meditsinkoe Izd, 1958 (in Russian).

Kavetskii, R. E., & Turkevich, N. Certain functional peculiarities of the pituitary and of the nervous system in mice of low and high and cancer strains. *Problems of Oncology*, 1959, *5*, 275-281.

Kelly, D. H., & Walters, C. J. The relationship between chemical diagnosis and anxiety, assessed by forearm blood flow and other measurements. *British Journal of Psychiatry*, 1968, *114*, 116-626.

Kerr, T. A., Schapira, K., & Roth, M. The relationship between premature death and affective disorders. *British Journal of Psychiatry,* 1969, *115,* 1277-1282.

Khaletskaia, F. M. Effect of overloading of the nervous system on the development of induced neoplasms in mice. *Zhurnal Vysshei Nervnoi Deiate L'nosti,* 1954, *4,* 869-876. (in Russian)

Khayetsky, I. K. Development of induced tumors under conditions of various effects on the hypothalamus. Symposium on genesis and hormonotherapy of cancer of the breast. Kiev, USSR, 1966.

Khinchin, A. *Mathematical foundations of information theory.* New York: Dover, 1957.

Kinsman, R. A., Spector, S. L., Shucard, D. W., & Luparello, T. J. Observations on patterns of subjective symptomatology of acute asthma. *Psychosomatic Medicine,* 1974, *36,* 129-143.

Kish, G. B. Studies of sensory reinforcement. In W. K. Honig (Ed.), *Operant behavior.* New York: Prentice-Hall, 1966.

Kish, G. B., & Busse, W. Correlates of stimulus seeking—Age, education, intelligence, and aptitudes. *Journal of Consulting & Clinical Psychology,* 1968, *32,* 633-637.

Kissen, D. M. Personality characteristics in males conducive to lung cancer. *British Journal of Medical Psychology,* 1963, *36,* 27-36.

Kissen, D. M. Personal communication to C. B. Bahnson, 1968. In C. B. Bahnson (Ed.), Dedication. In memory of Dr. David M. Kissen: his work and his thinking, *Annals of the New York Academy of Science,* 1969, *164,* 316.

Kissen, D. M. Relationship between lung cancer, cigarette smoking, inhalation and personality. *British Journal of Medical Psychology,* 1964, *37,* 203-216.

Kissen, D. M. Relationship between primary lung cancer and peptic ulcer in males. *Psychosomatic Medicine,* 1962, *24,* 133-147.

Kissen, D. M. The significance of personality in lung cancer in men. *Annals of the New York Academy of Sciences,* 1965b, *125,* 820-826.

Kissen, D. M. The value of a psychosomatic approach to cancer. *Annals of the New York Academy of Sciences,* 1965a, *125,* 777-779.

Kissen, D. M., & Eysenck, H. J. Personality in male lung cancer patients. *Journal of Psychosomatic Research,* 1962, *6,* 123-127.

Kissen, D. M., & LeShan, L. L. (Eds.). *Psychosomatic aspects of neoplastic disease.* J. B. Lippincott Co., 1964.

Kissen, D. M., & Rao, L. G. Steroid excretion patterns and personality in lung cancer. *Annals of the New York Academy of Science,* 1969, *164,* 476-482.

Klein, G. Tumor antigens. *Annual Review of Microbiology,* 1966, *20,* 223-252.

Knopp, W., Arnold, L. E., Smeltzer, D. J., and Andras, B. S. Pupillary light reaction as a predictor of amphetamine response in hyperkinetic children. *Psychopharmacology,* 1972, *26,* 53.

Koch, E. B. Die irradiation der pressoreceptorischen Kreislaufreflexe. *Klinische Wochenshrift,* 1932, *11,* 225-227.

Koestler, A. *The ghost in the machine.* New York: Macmillan, 1967.

Kollar, E. J. Psychological stress—a re-evaluation. *Journal of Nervous and Mental Disease,* 1961, *132,* 382-396.

Korneva, E. A., & Khai, L. M. Effect of destruction of areas of the hypothalamic region on the process of immunogenesis, *Fiziologicheskii Zhurnal SSSR,* 1963, *49,* 42-48.

Korneva, E. A. The effect of stimulating different mesencephalic structures on protective immune response patterns. *Fiziologicheskii Zhurnal SSSR,* 1967, *53,* 42-47.

Koroljow, S. Two cases of malignant tumors with metastases apparently treated successfully with hypoglycemic coma. *Psychiatric Quarterly,* 1962, *36,* 261-270.

Korschelt, R. *Lebensdanes, alten und tod.* Jena: Fischer, 1924.

Kowal, S. J. Emotions as cause of cancer: eighteenth and nineteenth century contributions. *Psychoanalytic Review,* 1955, *42,* 217-227.

Kruger, S., Robinson, G., & Scheuler, F. A study of the antileukemic activity of rauwolfia alkaloids. *Archives Internationales de Pharmacodynamie et de Therapie,* 1960, *129,* 125-130.

Kruger, S., Standeffer, W., & Schuler, F. Some aspects of reserpine on normal and leukemic mice. *Archives Internationales de Pharmacodynamie et de Therapie,* 1960, *129,* 345-400.

Kuhn, T. S. *The structure of scientific revolutions.* Chicago: University of Chicago Press, 1962.

Kupfer, D. J., & Foster, F. G. Interval between onset of sleep and rapid eye movement sleep as an indicator of depression. *Lancet,* 1972, *2,* 684-686.

Kutsky, R. J. *Handbook of vitamins and hormones.* New York: Van Nostrand Reinhold, 1973, p. 78.

LaBarba, R. C., & White, J. L. Maternal deprivation and the response to Ehrlich carcinoma in BALB/c mice. *Psychosomatic Medicine,* 1971, *33,* 458-460.

La Barba, R. C. Experiential and environmental factors in cancer. *Psychosomatic Medicine,* 1970, *32,* 259-276.

La Barba, R. C., White, J., & Lazar, J., et al. Early maternal separation and the response to Ehrlich carcinoma in BALB/c mice. *Developmental Psychology,* 1970, *3,* 78-80.

La Barba, R. C., Martini, J., & White, J. The effect of maternal separation on the growth of Ehrlich carcinoma in the BALB/c mouse. *Psychosomatic Medicine,* 1969, *31,* 129-133.

La Barba, R. C., Klein, M., White, J. L. The effects of early cold stress and handling on the growth of Ehrlich carcinoma in BALB/c mice. *Developmental Psychology,* 1970, *2,* 312-313.

Lacassagne, A. M. Apparition de cancers de la mamelle chez la souris male, soumise a des injections de folliculine. *Comptes Rendus, Academie des Sciences,* 1932, *195,* 630-632.

Lacassagne, A. Hypothalamus et cancer. *Presse Medicale,* 1961, *69,* 2285-2288.

Lacey, B. C., & Lacey, J. I. Studies of heart rate and other bodily processes in sensorimotor behavior. In P. A. Obrist (Ed.), *Cardio-*

vascular Psychophysiology. Chicago: Aldine, 1974, 538-564.

Lacey, J. I. Somatic response patterning and stress: some revisions of activation theory. In M. H. Appley & R. Trumball (Eds.), *Psychological stress: issues in research.* New York: Appleton-Century-Crofts, 1967, 14.

Lacey, J. I., Kagen, J., Lacey, B. C., & Moss, H. A. The visceral level: situational determinants and behavioral correlates of autonomic response patterns. In P. H. Knapp (Ed.), *Expression of the emotions in man.* New York: International Universities Press, 1963, 161-196.

Lader, M. H., and Wing, L. Physiological measures in agitated and retarded depressed patients. *Journal of Psychiatric Research,* 1969, 7, 89-100.

Lader, M., & Noble, P. The affective disorders. In P. H. Venables & M. J. Christie (Eds.), *Research in psychophysiology.* New York: John Wiley & Sons, 1975, 258-281.

Lang, P. J., & Buss, A. H. Psychological deficit in schizophrenia, II (Interference and activation). *Journal of Abnormal Psychology,* 1965, 70, 77-106.

Langworthy, O. R., & Richter, C. P. Increased spontaneous behavior produced by frontal lobe lesions in cats. *American Journal of Physiology,* 1939, 126, 158-161.

Larsen, J. K., Lindberg, M. L., & Skovgaard, B. Sleep deprivation as treatment for endogenous depression. *Acta Psychiatrica Scandinavica,* 1976, 54, 167-173.

Laszlo, E. *The systems view of the world.* New York: Braziller, 1972.

Lauber, H. L. Sexualle enthemmung und exhibitionismus bei frontal hirnverletzen. *Archives Psychiatrie Zeitschrift gesand Neurologie,* 1958, 197, 293-306.

Lawrence, D. H. The nature of a stimulus: some relationships between learning and perception. In S. Koch (Ed.), *Psychology: A study of a science (Vol. 5).* New York: McGraw-Hill, 1963, 179-212.

Lawrence, J. C. Gastrointestinal polyps—statistical study of malignancy incidence. *American Journal of Surgery,* 1936, 31, 499-505.

Lemieux, G., Davigon, A., & Genest, J. Depressive states during Rauwolfia therapy for arterial hypertension: a report of 30 cases. *Canadian Medical Association Journal,* 1956, 74, 522-526.

Lemonde, P. Influence of fighting on leukemia in mice. *Proceedings of the Society for Experimental Biology and Medicine,* 1959, 102, 292-295.

Lemonde, P. Inhibition of experimental leukemia by a combination of various factors. *Lancet,* 1966, 2, 946-947.

LeShan, L. A basic psychological orientation apparently associated with malignant disease. *Psychiatric Quarterly,* 1961, 35, 314-339.

LeShan, L. An emotional life-history pattern associated with neoplastic disease. *Annals of the New York Academy of Sciences,* 1965, 125, 780-793.

LeShan, L. The personality of cancer patients: an interim report. Paper presented at the convention of the American Psychological Association, Sept. 1962, Philadelphia, Pennsylvania.

LeShan, L. Psychological states as factors in the development of malignant disease: a critical review. *Journal of the National Cancer Institute,* 1959, *22,* 1-18.

LeShan, L., & Reznikoff, M. A psychological factor apparently associated with neoplastic disease. *Journal of Abnormal and Social Psychology,* 1960, *60,* 439-440.

LeShan, L., & Worthington, R. E. Some recurrent life history patterns observed in patients with malignant disease. *Journal of Nervous and Mental Disease,* 1956, *124,* 460-465.

Lester, B. K., Chanes, R. E., & Condit, P. T. A clinical syndrome and EEG-sleep changes associated with amino acid deprivation. *The American Journal of Psychiatry,* 1969, *126,* 185-190.

Leuba, C. Toward some integration of learning theories—the concept of optimal stimulation. *Psychological Reports,* 1955, *1,* 27-33.

Leuba, C. Relation of stimulation intensities to learning and development. *Psychological Reports,* 1962, *11,* 55-56.

Levey, R. H., & Medawar, P. B. Some experiments on the action of antilymphoid antisera. *Annals of the New York Academy of Sciences,* 1966, *129,* 164-177.

Levin H., & Forgays D. G. Learning as a function of sensory stimulation of various intensities. *Journal of Comparative and Physiological Psychology,* 1959, *52,* 195-201.

Levine, S., & Cohen, C. Differential survival to leukemia as a function of infantile stimulation in DBA/2 mice. *Proceedings of the Society for Experimental Biology and Medicine,* 1959, *120,* 53-54.

Levine, S. Psychophysiological effects of infantile stimulation. In E. L. Bliss (Ed.), *Roots of behavior.* New York: Harper & Row, 1962, 246.

Lewis, M. R., & Cole, W. H. Experimental increase of lung metastases after operative trauma (amputation of limb with tumor). *Archives of Surgery,* 1958, *77,* 621.

Lewis, N. D. C. *Research in dementia præcox (Past attainments, present trends and future possibilities).* New York: National Committee for Mental Hygiene, 1936.

Li, F. P., & Fraumeni, J. F. Rhabdomyosarcoma in children—Epidemiologic study and identification of a familial cancer syndrome. *Journal of the National Cancer Insitute,* 1969a, *43,* 1365-1373.

Li, F. P., & Fraumeni, J. F. Soft-tissue sarcomas, breast cancer, and other neoplasms—a familial syndrome? *Annals of Internal Medicine,* 1969b, *71,* 747-752.

Li, F. P., Rapoport, A. H., Fraumeni, J. F., & Jenson, R. D. Familial ovarian carcinoma. *Journal of the American Medical Association,* 1970, *214,* 1559-1561.

Lifton, R. From analysis to form: towards a shift in psychological paradigm. *Salmagundi*, 1975, *28*, 43-78.

Lindsley, D. B.   Common factors in sensory deprivation, sensory distortion, and sensory overload. In P.   Solomon et al (Eds.), *Sensory deprivation.* Cambridge, Massachusetts: Harvard University Press, 1961, 174-194.

Lindsley, D. B.   Emotion.   In S. S. Stevens (Ed.), *Handbook of experimental psychology.* New York: John Wiley & Sons, 1951, p. 473.

Lindsley, D. B.   Psychophysiology and motivation. In Jones, M. R. (Ed.), *Nebraska symposium on motivation.* Lincoln: University of Nebraska Press, 1957, 44-105.

Loeser, A.   A new therapy for prevention of post-operative recurrences in genital and breast cancer.   *British Medical Journal*, 1954, *2*, 1380-1383.

Lord Brain, Wilkinson M.   Subacute cerebellar degeneration associated with neoplasms. *Brain*, 1965, *88*, 465-478.

Ludwig, A. M.   Self-regulation of the sensory environment.   *Archives of General Psychiatry*, 1971, *25*, 413-418.

Ludwig, A. M.   "Psychedelic" effects produced by sensory overload. *American Journal of Psychiatry*, 1972, *128*, 1294-1297.

Lugaresi, E., Coccagna, G., Ceroni, G. B., Gambi, D., & Poppi, M.   Restless legs syndrome and nocturnal myoclonus. In H. Gastaut et al (Eds.), *The abnormalities of sleep in man.* Proceedings of the Twenty-fifth European meeting on Electroencephalography, Bologna, 1967, 285.

Luria, A. R.   Disorders of simultaneous perception in a case of bilateral occipitoparietal brain injury. *Brain*, 1959, *82*, 437-449.

Luria, A. R., Karpov B. A., & Yarbus A. L.   Disturbance of active visual perception with lesions of the frontal lobes. *Cortex*, 1966, *2*, 202-212.

Lynn, R.   *Attention, arousal, and the orientation reaction.* Elmsford, New York: Pergamon Press, 1966.

Mabry, P. D., & Campbell, B. A.   Ontogeny of serotonergic inhibition of behavioral arousal in the rat.   *Journal of Comparative and Physiological Psychology*, 1974, *86*, 193-201.

Mackenzie, I., & Rous, P.   The experimental disclosure of latent neoplastic changes in tarred skin.   *Journal of Experimental Medicine*, 1941, *73*, 391-415.

Madigan, F. C., & Vance, R. B. Differential sex mortality: a research design. *Social Forces*, 1957, *35*, 193-199.

Maliugina, L. L., Mironova, A. I., Fedorov, V. K., & Shabad, L. M. The significance of higher nervous activity in the appearance and development of tumors of the breast in mice.   *Bulletin of Experimental Biology and Medicine*, 1958, *45*, 727-731.

Malmo, R. B.   Activation—a neurophysiological dimension. *Psychological Review*, 1959, *66*, 367-386.

Marchant, J.   The effect of methlcholanthrene and different social conditions on the appearance of breast tumors in NZY mice. *British Journal of Cancer*, 1966, *20*, 210-215.

Marchant, J. The effects of different social conditions on breast cancer induction in three genetic types of mice by dibenz(a,h)anthracene and a comparison with breast carcinoma by 3-methylcholanthrene. *British Journal of Cancer,* 1967, *21,* 576-585.

Marcus, M. G. Cancer and character. *Psychology Today,* 1976, *10,* 52-60.

Mark, V. H., & Ervin, F. R. *Violence and the brain.* New York: Harper & Row, 1970.

Marsh, G. R., & Thompson, L. W. Psychophysiology of aging. In J. E. Birren, & K. W. Schaie (Eds.), *Handbook of the psychology of aging.* New York: Van Nostrand Reinhold, 1977, 219.

Marsh, J. T., Lavender, J. F., Shueh-Shen, C., & Rasmussen, A. F. Poliomyelitis in monkeys—Decreased susceptibility after avoidance stress. *Science,* 1963, *140,* 1414-1415.

Marsh, J. T., Miller, B. E., & Lamson, B. G. Effect of repeated brief stress on growth of Ehrlich carcinoma in the mouse. *Journal of the National Cancer Institute,* 1959, *22,* 961-977.

Matthes, T. Experimental contribution to the question of emotional stress reactions on the growth of tumors in animals. *Acta Unio Contra Cancrum,* 1964, *20,* 1608-1610.

McCance, R. A. Characteristics of the newly born. In G. E. W. Wolstenholme & M. O'Connor (Eds.), *Somatic stability in the newly born.* Boston: Little, Brown & Co., 1961, 1-4.

McGinty, D. J., Arand, D. L. & Littner, M. R. Sleep-related breathing disorders in healthy and hypersomnolent older males. Paper read at APSS Annual Meeting, Hyannis, Massachusetts, June 1981.

McGinty, D. J., London, M.S., & Stevenson, M. Effects of rocking bed on breathing during sleep in kittens. Paper presented at Annual Meeting of APSS, Hyannis, Massachusetts, June 1981.

McGrady, P. *The savage cell.* New York: Basic Books, 1964, 21.

Mednick, S. A. Autonomic nervous system recovery and psychopathology. *Scandinavian Journal of Behavior Therapy,* 1975, *4,* 55-68.

McKinlay, J. B., & McKinlay, S. M. The questionable contribution of medical measures to the decline of mortality in the United States in the twentieth century. In S. J. Williams (Ed.), *Issues in health services.* New York: John Wiley & Sons, 1980, 3-16.

Mekhedova, A. Vozniknovenie nevroticheskikh sostoianii u sobak pri zamene postoiannogo podkrepleniia uslovnykh signalov veroiasnostym. *Zhurnal Vysshei Nervnoi Deiatelnosti,* 1974, *24,* 243-251.

Meerloo, A. M. The initial neurologic and psychiatric picture syndrome of pulmonary growth. *Journal of the American Medical Association,* 1944, *126,* 558-559.

Meerloo, A. M. Psychological implications of malignant growth: survey of hypotheses. *British Journal of Medical Psychology,* 1954, *27,* 210-215.

Meerloo, A. M., & Zeckel, A. Psychiatric problems of malignancy. In L. Bellak (Ed.), *Psychology of physical illness.* New York: Grune and Stratton, 1952, 45-51.

Mellett, P. The birth of asthma. *Journal of Psychosomatic Research,* 1978, *22,* 239-246.

Michel, F., Jeannerod, M., Mouret, J., Rechtschaffen, A., & Jouvet, M. Sur les mecanismes de l'activite de pointes au niveau du systeme visuel au cours de la phase paradoxale du sommeil. *Comptes Rendus des Seances de la Societe de Biologie et de ses Filiales,* 1964, *158,* 103-106.

Miller, F. R., & Jones, H. W. The possibility of precipitating the leukemic state by emotional factors. *Blood, Journal of Hematology,* 1948, *3,* 880-884.

Miller, G. A. The magical number seven, plus or minus two! *Psychological Review,* 1956, *63,* 81-97.

Miller, G. A., Galanter, E., & Pribram, K. H. *Plans and the structure of behavior.* New York: Holt, Rinehart & Winston, 1960.

Miller, J. A. Carcinogenesis by chemicals—an overview—G. H. A. Clowes Memorial Lecture. *Cancer Research,* 1970, *30,* 559-576.

Miller, J. A., & Miller, E. C. The carcinogenic aminoazo dyes. *Advances in Cancer Research,* 1953, *1,* 339-396.

Miller, J. F. A. P. Immunological function of the thymus. *Lancet,* 1961, *2,* 748-749.

Miller, J. G. Information input overload and psychopathology. *American Journal of Psychiatry,* 1960, *116,* 695-704.

Miller, J. G. Living systems. *The Quarterly Review of Biology,* 1973, *48,* 63-276.

Mirsky, A. F. The neuropsychological basis of schizophrenia. *Annual Review of Psychology,* 1969, *20,* 321-348.

Mirsky, I. A. Physiologic, psychologic, and social determinants in the etiology of duodenal ulcer. *American Journal of Digestive Diseases,* 1958, *3,* 285-314.

Mischel, W. *Personality and assessment.* New York, John Wiley & Sons, 1968.

Mischel, W. Toward a cognitive social learning reconceptualization of personality. *Psychological Review,* 1973, *80,* 252-283.

Modan, B., Lubin, F., Barell, V., Greenberg, R. A., Modan, M., & Graham, S. The role of starches in the etiology of gastric cancer. *Cancer* (Philadelphia), 1974, *34,* 2087-2092.

Molinari, S., & Foulkes, D. Tonic and phasic events during sleep: psychological correlates and implications. *Perceptual and Motor Skills,* 1969, *29,* 343-368 (Monograph Supplement I-V29).

Molkov, I. V. N. Effect of biopsy and of injuries of the skin on cell division in tumors (Translated title). *Voprosy Onkologii,* 1955, *1* (2), 3-7.

Monjan, A. A., & Collector, M. I. Stress-induced modulation of the immune response. *Science,,* 1977, *196,* 307-308.

Moorcroft, W. H., Lytle, L. D., & Campbell, B. A. Ontogeny of starvation-induced behavioral arousal in the rat. *Journal of Comparative and Physiological Psychology,* 1971, *75,* 59-67.

Morton, D. L., Haskell, C. M., Pilch, Y. H., Sparkes, F. C., & Winters, W. D. Recent advances in oncology. *Annals of Internal*

Medicine, 1972, *77,* 431-454.

Moser, R. H. Knowledge is not enough. *New England Journal of Medicine,* 1977, *296,* 938-940.

Muhlbock, O. Influence of environment on the incidence of mammary tumors in mice. *Acta Unio Internationalis Contra Cancrum,* 1950, *7,* 351-353.

Munro, A. Parental deprivation in depressive patients. *British Journal of Psychiatry,* 1966, *112,* 443-457.

Muses, C. Hypernumber and metadimension theory. *Journal for the Study of Consciousness,* 1968, *1,* 30-48.

Muslin, H. L., Gyarfas, K., & Pieper, W. J. Separation experience and cancer of the breast. *Annals of the New York Academy of Sciences,* 1966, *125,* 801-806.

Naranjo, C., and Ornstein, R. *On the psychology of meditation.* New York: Viking Press, 1971.

Neisser, U. *Cognitive psychology.* New York: Prentice-Hall, 1967.

Nesterova-Kozhevnikova, E. P. *On the change in tissue respiration and glycolysis and the role of higher nervous activity in the experimental formation of tumors.* Doctoral dissertation, Sverdlovsk, USSR, 1951.

von Neumann, J. *The computer and the brain.* New Haven: Yale University Press, 1958.

von Neumann, J. *Mathematical foundations of quantum mechanics.* Princeton: Princeton University Press, 1955.

Newberry, B. H., Frankie, G., Beatty, P. A., Maloney, B. D., & Gilchrist, J. C. Shock stress and DMBA—induced mammary tumors. *Psychosomatic Medicine,* 1972, *34,* 295-303.

Newberry, B. H., Gildow, J., Wogan, J., & Reese, R. L. Inhibition of Huggins tumors by forced restraint. *Psychosomatic Medicine,* 1976, *38,* 155-162.

Newton, G. Early experience and resistance to tumor growth. In D. M. Kissen & L. L. LeShan (Eds.), *Psychosomatic aspects of neoplastic disease.* Philadelphia: J. B. Lippincott Co., 1964, p. 71.

Newton, G. Tumor susceptibility in rats—Role of infantile manipulation and later exercise. *Psychological Reports,* 1965, *16,* 127-132.

Newton, G., Bly, C. G., & McCrary, C. Effects of early experience on the response to transplanted tumors. *Journal of Nervous and Mental Disorders,* 1962, *134,* 522-527.

Nikitina, G. M. Correlations in the development of orientation and conditioned motor reactions in ontogenesis. *Zhurnal Vysshei Nervnoi Deiatel'Nosti Imene I. P. Pavlova,* 1954, *4,* 406-414.

Nix, J. T. Study of the relationship of environmental factors to the type and frequency of cancer causing death in nuns. *Hospital Progress,* 1964, *45,* 71-74.

Nobel, K. W., & Dewson, J. H., III. A corticofugal projection from insular and temporal cortex to the homolateral inferior colliculus in cat. *Journal of Auditory Research,* 1966, *6,* 67-75.

Noble, P., & Lader, M. The symptomatic correlates of skin conductance changes in depression. *Journal of Psychiatric Research,* 1971, *9,* 61-69.

Nunn, T. W. *On cancer of the breast.* London, England: Churchill, 1882

Olenov, Y. M. On induced cancer in mice with experimental neurosis. *Voprosi Onkologii* (Leningrad), 1955, *8,* 26-32.

Ornitz, E. M., Wechter, V., Hartman, D., Tanguay, P. E., Lee, C. M., Ritvo, E., R., & Walter, R. D. The EEG and rapid eye movements during REM sleep in babies. *Electroencephalography and Clinical Neurophysiology,* 1971, *30,* 350-353.

Ornstein, R. *The Psychology of Consciousness.* San Francisco: W. H. Freeman, 1972.

Orr, W. C. Is a good night's sleep really good? Paper read at Annual meeting of Society for Psychophysiological Research, Cincinnati, Ohio, 1979.,

Oswald, I. Falling asleep open-eyed during intense rhythmic stimulation. *British Medical Journal,* 1960, *1,* 1450-1455.

Oswald, I. *Sleeping and waking: physiology and psychology.* Amsterdam and New York: Elsevier, 1962.

Otis, L. S., & Scholler, J. Effects of stress during infancy on tumor development and tumor growth. *Psychological Reports,* 1967, *20,* 167-173.

Owens, W. A. Is age kinder to the initially more able? *Journal of Gerontology,* 1959, *14,* 334-337.

Paget, I. *Surgical pathology.* Second edition. London, England: Longmans Green, 1870.

Paloucek, F. P., & Graham, J. B. Precipitating factors in cancer of the cervix. *Surgical Forum,* 1960, *10,* 740-742.

Pare, W. R. Age, sex, and strain differences in the aversive threshold to grid shock in the rat. *Journal of Comparative and Physiological Psychology,* 1969, *69,* 214-218.

Parkes, C. M., Benjamin, B., & Fitzgerald, R. G. Broken heart: a statistical study of increased mortality among widowers. *British Medical Journal,* 1969, *1,* 740-743.

Pattee, H. H., & Waddington, C. H. (Eds.), *Towards a theoretical biology.* (Prolegomena), (Vol. 1). Chicago: Aldine, 1967.

Pearson, O. H., Llerena, O., Llerena, L., et al. Prolactin-dependent rat mammary cancer—a model for man. *Transactions of the Association of American Physicians,* 1969, *32,* 225-237.

Peller, S. *Quantitative research in human biology and medicine.* Bristol, England: John Wright & Sons, 1967.

Pelletier, K. R. *Toward a science of consciousness.* New York: Delacorte Press, 1978.

Pelletier, K. R. *Holistic medicine: from pathology to optimum health.* New York: Delacorte Press, 1979.

Perrin, G. M., & Pierce, I. R. Psychosomatic aspects of cancer. *Psychosomatic Medicine,* 1959, *21,* 397-421.

Perry, J. W. Reconstitutive process in the psychotherapy of the self. *Annals of the New York Academy of Science,* 1962, *96,* 853-876.

Peters, L. J., & Mason, K. A. Influence of stress on experimental cancer. In B. A. Stoll (Ed.), *Mind and cancer prognosis.* New York: John Wiley & Sons, 1979, 103-124.

Petre-Quadens, O., de Lee, C., & Remy, M. Eye movement density during sleep and brain maturation. *Brain Research,* 1971, *26,* 49-56.

Petre-Quadens, O., & de Lee, C. Eye movements during sleep: a common criterion of learning capacities and endocrine activity. *Developmental Medicine and Child Neurology,* 1970, *12,* 730-740.

Petrinovich, L. Probabilistic functionalism: a conception of research method. *American Psychologist,* 1979, *34,* 373-390.

Petrova, M. K. *On the role of functionally weakened cerebral cortex in the origin of various pathological processes.* Moscow: Medgiz, 1946.

Petrovoskii, I. N. Problems of nervous control in immunity reactions—II—the influence of experimental neuroses on immunity reactions. *Zhurnal Mikrobiologii, Epidemiologii I Immunobiologii,* 1961, *32,* 1411 ff.

Piaget, J. *The origins of intelligence in children.* New York: International Universities Press, 1952.

Piaget, J. *Structuralism.* New York: Harper & Row, 1970.

Piaget, J. What is psychology? *American Psychologist,* 1978, *33,* 648-652.

Pitot, H. C., & Heidelberger, C. Metabolic regulatory circuits and carcinogenesis. *Cancer Research,* 1963, *23,* 1694-1700.

Plum, H. F. *Carcinogenesis by ultraviolet light.* Princeton, New Jersey: Princeton University Press, 1959.

Polanyi, M. Life transcending physics and chemistry. *Chemical Engineering News,* 1967, *45,* 54-66.

Polanyi, M. *The tacit dimension.* New York: Doubleday & Co., 1966.

Polednak, A. P. College athletics, body size and cancer mortality. *Cancer,* 1976, *38,* 382-387.

Popper, K. R., Three views concerning human knowledge. In H. D. Lewis (Ed.), *Contemporary British philosophy.* London: Allen and Union, 1956.

Potter, W., & Heron, W. Sleep during perceptual deprivation. *Brain Research,* 1972, *40,* 534-539.

Powers, W. T. *Behavior—the control of perception.* Chicago: Aldine Publishing Company, 1973.

Pratt, K. C. The neonate. In L. Carmichael (Ed.), *Manual of child psychology.* New York: John Wiley & Sons, 1946.

Prechtl, H. F. R., & Lenard, H. G. A study of eye movements in sleeping newborn infants. *Brain Research,* 1967, *5,* 477-493.

Prehn, R. T. Immunosurveillance, regeneration and oncogenesis. *Progress in Experimental Tumor Research,* 1971, *14,* 1-24.

Prentsky, R. A. Creativity and psychopathology: a neurocognitive perspective. In B. A. Maher (Ed.), *Progress in experimental personality research.* New York: Academic Press, 1979, 1-39.

Prevost, F., De Koninck, J., Barry, W. et al. Inversion of the visual field and REM sleep: experimental reconciliation of the P-hypothesis and the SCIP-hypothesis. *Sleep Research,* 1974, *3,* 89.

Prevost, F., De Koninck, J., & Prouix, G. Stage REM rapid eye movements following visual inversion: further investigation and replication. *Sleep Research,* 1975, *4,* 57.

Pribram, K. Personal communication, 1969.

Pribram, K. H. The new neurology and the biology of emotion: a structural approach. *American Psychologist,* 1967, *22,* 830-838.

Pribram, K. H. Problems concerning the structure of consciousness. In G. Globus (Ed.), *Brain and conscious experience.* New York: Plenum, 1976.

Pribram, K. H., & Melges, F. T. Psychophysiological basis of emotion. In P. Vinken & G. Bruyn (Eds.) *Handbook of clinical neurology.* Amsterdam: North Holland Publishing Co., 1969, 316-342.

Puzhak, H. Y. On the importance of the sympathico-adrenal system in the regulation of the mitotic activity in normal and tumor tissues in the white rat. *Acta Unio Internationalis Cancrum,* 1974, *20,* 1621-1622.

Quay, H. C. Psychopathic personality as pathologic stimulation-seeking. *American Journal of Psychiatry,* 1966, *122,* 180-183.

Quadri, S., Kledzik, G., & Meites, J. Effects of L-dopa and methyldopa on growth of mammary cancers in rats. *Proceedings of the Society of Experimental Biology and Medicine,* 1973, *142,* 759-761.

Rauf, Y. Psychosomatic aspects of cancer reasearch. *National Federation of Spiritual Healers.* (date unknown).

Ramey, E. R. Boredom: the most prevalent American disease. *Harper's,* November, 1974, 12-22.

Rashkis, H. A. Systemic stress as an inhibitor of experimental tumors in Swiss mice. *Science,* 1952, *116,* 169-171.

Rasmussen, A. F., Marsh, J. T., & Brill, N. Q. Increased susceptibility to Herpes simplex in mice subjected to avoidance-learning stress or restraint. *Proceedings of the Society for Experimental Biology and Medicine,* 1957, *96,* 183-189.

Raushenbakh, M., Zharova, E., & Khakhlova, M. The influence of overstraining of the central nervous system in mice on the development of experimental leukocytosis. *Arkhiv Patologii,* 1952, *14,* 23-31. (in Russian)

Ray, P., & Pradhan, S. N. Growth of transplanted and induced tumors in rats under a schedule of punished behavior. *Journal of the National Cancer Institute,* 1974, *52,* 575-577.

Rechtschaffen, A., & Monroe, L. Laboratory studies of insomnia. In A. Kales (Ed.), *Sleep: physiology and pathology,* Philadelphia: J. B. Lippincott Co., 1969, 158.

Rechtschaffen, A., Verdone, P., & Wheaton, J. Reports of mental activity during sleep. *Canadian Psychiatric Association Journal,* 1963, *8,* 409-414.

Reznikoff, M. Psychological factors in breast cancer: A preliminary study of some personality trends in patients with cancer of the breast. *Psychosomatic Medicine,* 1955, *17,* 96-108.

Reznikoff, M., & Martin, D. E. The influence of stress on mammary cancer in mice. *Journal of Psychosomatic Research,* 1958, *2,* 56-60.

Richards, V. *Cancer - the wayward cell—its origins, nature and treatment.* Berkeley: University of California Press, 1972.

Richter, D. The stability of the nervous system during development. In G. E. W. Wolstenholme & M. O'Connor (Eds.), *Somatic stability in the newly born.* Boston: Little, Brown & Co., 1961, 306-310.

Riley, V. Mouse mammary tumors: alteration of incidence as apparent function of stress. *Science,* 1975, *189,* 465-467.

Robinson, R. *Tumours that secrete catecholamines: their detection and clinical chemistry.* New York: John Wiley & Sons, 1980.

Røjel, J. The interrelationship between uterine cancer and syphilis—a patho-demographic study. *Acta Pathologica et Microbiologica Scandinavia Supplement,* 1953, *97,* 3-82.

Roffo, A. H. Uber die physikalisch—chemische aetiology der krebskrankheit. *Strahlentherapie,* 1939, *66,* 328-350.

Roffwarg, H. P. Diagnostic classification of sleep and arousal disorders. *Sleep,,* 1979, *2,* 1-15.

Roffwarg, H. P., Muzio, J. N., & Dement, W. C. Ontogenetic development of the human sleep-dream cycle. *Science,* 1966, *152,* 604-619.

Rollin, B. *First you cry.* Philadelphia: J. B. Lippincott Co., 1974.

Ross, W. C. J. The chemistry of cytotoxic alkylating agents. *Advances in Cancer Research,* 1953, *1,* 397-449.

Royal, R. Study cited in W. C. Dement, *Some must watch while some must sleep.* San Francisco: San Francisco Book Company, 1976, 15.

Ruddon, R. W. *Cancer biology.* New York: Oxford University Press, 1981, 213-222.

Rusch, H. P., & Kline, B. E. The effect of exercise on the growth of a mouse tumor. *Cancer Research,* 1944, *4,* 116-118.

Rush, B. F. Rational approach to the therapy of primary breast cancer. Lecture in a course, "Topics in clinical oncology: breast carcinoma." American College of Physicians, 1975.

Ryback, R. S., & Lewis, O. F. Effects of prolonged bed rest on EEG sleep patterns in young, healthy volunteers. *Electroencephalography and Clinical Neurophysiology,* 1971, *31,* 395-399.

Saffioti, U., Montesano, R., Sellakumar, A. R., & Borg, S. A. Experimental cancer of the lung. Inhibition by vitamin A of the induction of tracheobronchial squamous metaplasia and squamous cell tumors. *Cancer,* 1967, *20,* 857-864.

Saint-Hilaire, S., Lavers, M. K., Kennedy, J., & Code, C. F. Gastric acid secretory value of different foods. *Gastroenterology,* 1960, *39,* 1-11.

Samundzhan, E. M. Effect of functionally weakened cerebral cortex on growth of inoculated tumors in mice. *Meditsinskaia Zhurnal,* 1954, *24,* 10-14.

Sanford, K. K., Earle, W. R., Shelton E., Schilling, E. L., Duchesne, E. M., Likely, G. D., & Becker, M. M. Production of malignancy in vitro—XII—Further transformations of mouse fibroblasts to sarcomatous cells. *Journal of the National Cancer Institute,* 1950, *11,* 351-367.

Sarfatti, J. The physical roots of consciousness. In J. Mishlove (Ed.) *The roots of consciousness.* New York: Random House, 1975.

Satterfield, J. H., Cantwell, D. P., Lesser, L. I., & Podosin, R. L. Physiological studies of the hyperkinetic child: I. *The American Journal of Psychiatry,* 1972, *128,* 102-108.

Satterfield, J. H., & Dawson, M. E. Electrodermal correlates of hyperactivity in children. *Psychophysiology,* 1971, *8,* 191-197.

Saward, E., & Sorensen, A. The current emphasis on preventive medicine. In S. J. Williams (Ed.), *Issues in health services.* New York: John Wiley & Sons, 1980, 17-30.

Schaie, K. W., & Strother, C. R. *A cross-sequential study of age changes in cognitive behavior.* Paper presented at the meeting of the Midwestern Psychological Association, St. Louis, April, 1964.

Schalling, D. Psychopathic behavior: personality and neuropsychology. In R. D. Hare and D. Schalling (Eds.), *Psychopathic behavior: approaches to research.* Chichester: John Wiley & Sons, 1978.

Schatten, W. E., & Kramer, W. M. An experimental study of postoperative tumor metastases. II. Effects of anesthesia, operation, and cortisone administration on growth of pulmonary metastases. *Cancer,* 1958, *11,* 460-462.

Scheflen, A. E. Malignant tumors in the institutionalized psychotic population. *Archives of Neurology and Psychiatry,* 1951, *66,* 145-155.

Schildkraut, J. J., & Kety, S. S. Biogenic amines and emotion. *Science,* 1967, *156,* 21-30.

Schlosberg, H. Three dimensions of emotion. *Psychological Review,* 1954, *61,* 81-88.

Schmale, A., & Iker, H. The psychological setting of uterine cervical cancer. *Annals of The New York Academy of Sciences,* 1965, *125,* 807-813.

Schmale, A. H., & Iker, H. P. The effect of hopelessness in the development of cancer. 1. The prediction of uterine cervical cancer in women with atypical cytology. *Psychosomatic Medicine,* 1964, *26,* 634-635.

Schmale, A. H., Jr. Relationship of separation and depression to disease. I. A report on a hospitalized medical population. *Psychosomatic Medicine,* 1958, *20,* 259-277.

Schneppenheim, P., Hamperl, H., & Kaufmann, C. Die beziehungen des schleimepithels zum plattenepithel an der cervix uteri im lebanslauf der frau. *Archiv für Gynakologie,* 1958, *190,* 303. (As shown by Hamperl, H., & Kaufmann, C. The cervix uteri at different ages. *Obstetrics and Gynecology*, 1959, *14*, 621-631.)

Schomig, G. Die weiblichen genitalkarzinome bei sexueller enthaltsamkeit. *Strahlentherapie*, 1953, *92*, 156-158.

Schroder, H. M., Driver, M. J., & Struefert, S. *Human information processing*. New York: Holt, Rinehart & Winston, 1967.

Schultz, D. P. (Ed.) *Sensory restriction—Effects on behavior*. New York: Academic Press, 1965.

Schwartz, D., Flamant, R., Lellouch, J., & Denoix, P. F. Results of a French survey on the role of tobacco, particularly inhalation, in different cancer sites. *Journal of the National Cancer Institute*, 1961, *26*, 1085-1108.

Schwartz, G. E. Psychobiological foundations of psychotherapy and behavior change. In S. L. Garfield & A. E. Bergin (Eds.), *Handbook of psychotherapy and behavior change.* New York: John Wiley & Sons, 1978, 63-99.

Schwartz, G. E. Psychosomatic disorders and biofeedback: a psychobiological model of disregulation. In J. D. Maser & M. E. Seligman (Eds.), *Psychopathology: experimental models.* San Francisco: W. H. Freeman & Co., 1977, 270-307.

Schwartz, G. E., & Weiss, S. M. Behavioral medicine revisited: an amended definition. *Journal of Behavioral Medicine*, 1978, *1*, 249-251.

Seidenburg, R. The trauma of eventlessness. In J. B. Miller (Ed.), *Psychoanalysis and women.* New York: Penguin Books, 1973.

Seifter, E., Retturg, G., Zisblatt, M., Levenson, S. M., Levine, N., Davidson, A., & Seifter, J. Enhancement of tumor development in physically-stressed mice inoculated with an oncogenic virus. *Experentia* (Basel), 1973, *29*, 1379-1382.

Selye, H. *Stress.* Montreal: ACTA Medical Publishers, 1950.

Selye, H. *The stress of life.* New York: McGraw-Hill, 1956.

Shands, H. C., Finesinger, J. E., Cobb, S., & Abrams, R. D. Psychological mechanisms in patients with cancer. *Cancer*, 1951, *4*, 1159-1170.

Shannon, C. E. A mathematical theory of communication. *Bell Systems Technology Journal*, 1948, *26*, 623-656.

Sharpless, S., & Jasper, H. H. Habituation of the arousal reaction. *Brain*, 1956, *79*, 655-680.

Shelton, E., Evans, V. J., & Parker, G. A. Malignant transformation of mouse connective tissue grown in diffusion chambers. *Journal of the National Cancer Institute*, 1963, *30*, 377-391.

Sherman, E. D., & Robillard, E. Sensitivity to pain in the aged. *Canadian Medical Association Journal*, 1960, *83*, 944-947.

Shevrin, H., & Dickman, S. The psychological unconscious: a necessary assumption for all psychological theory? *American Psychologist*, 1980, *35*, 421-434.

Shiffrin, R. M., & Schneider, W. Controlled and automatic information processing: II. Perceptual learning, automatic attending, and a general theory. *Psychological Review*, 1977, *84*, 127-190.

Silverman, J. A paradigm for the study of altered states of

consciousness. *British Journal of Psychiatry*, 1968, *114*, 1201-1218.

Silverman, J. Variations in cognitive control and psychophysiological defense in the schizophrenias. *Psychosomatic Medicine*, 1967, *29*, 225-251.

Silverstein, H., Lazere, F., Sandler, A., & Graves, S. Subconvulsive audiogenic stress effect on chemical carcinogenesis and transplanted tumors. *Federation Proceedings*, 1961, *20*, 326.

Silverstone, H. Skin cancer in Queensland, Australia. In H. F. Blum & F. Urbach (Eds.), *Report of the Airlie house conference on sunlight and skin cancer.* Bethesda: National Institutes of Health, 1964.

Sing-Mao, L. Effects of neurosis on appearance and development of induced mammary gland tumors in rats. *Federation Proceedings. Translation Supplement*, 1963, *22*, 1241-1244.

Sinha, D., & Dao, T. Estrogen and induction of mammary cancer. In T. L. Dao (Ed.), *Estrogen target tissues and neoplasia.* Chicago: University of Chicago Press, 1972, 307-316.

Smith, A. E., & Kenyon, D. H. A unifying concept of carcinogenesis and its therapeutic implications. *Oncology*, 1973, *27*, 459-479.

Smith, L. W., & Lazere, F. The effect of audiogenic stress upon the growth of methylcholanthrene induced tumors. *Federation Proceedings*, 1960, *19*, 384.

Smith, S., Myers, T. I., & Murphy, D. B. Restlessness and life-sustaining activities during four days of sensory deprivation. *Psychonomic Sciences*, 1967, *8*, 523-524.

Smithers, D. W. *Clinical prospect of the cancer problem.* London: Livingston, 1960.

Smyth, M., Giblin, E. C., & Lee, K. Prevalence of apneas and oxygen desaturation during sleep in healthy older men. Paper read at APSS Annual Meeting, Hyannis, Massachusetts, June 1981.

Snow, H. *A treatise, practical and theoretic, on cancers and the cancer process.* London: Churchill, 1893.

Snyder, F. Electroencephalographic studies of sleep in psychiatric disorders. In M. H. Chase (Ed.), *The sleeping brain.* Los Angeles Brain Research Institute, 1972, 376.

Snyder, F., Hobson, J. A., Morrison, P. F., and Goldfrank, F. Changes in respiration, heart rate, and systolic blood pressure in human sleep. *Journal of Applied Physiology*, 1964, *19*, 417-422.

Sokolov, E. H. Neuronal models and the orienting reflex. In M. A. B. Brazier (Ed.), *The central nervous system and behavior.* New York: Josiah Macy, Jr. Foundation, 1960, 187.

Solomon, G. F. Stress and antibody response in rats. *International Archives of Allergy and Applied Immunology*, 1969, *35*, 97-104.

Somogyi, A., & Kovacs, K. Effect of stress on the adrenocorticolytic and carcinogenic action of 7, 12, dimethylbenz(a)anthracene. *Zeitschrift für Krebsforschung*, 1971, *75*, 288-295.

Southam, C. M., Moore, A. E., & Rhoads, C. P. Homotransplantation of human cell lines. *Science*, 1957, *125*, 158-160.

Sparks, A. K. Tumors and tumor-like conditions in invertebrates. In A. K. Sparks (Ed.), *Invertebrate pathology—Noncommunicable diseases*. New York: Academic Press, 1972, 274-367.

Sparks, A. K. Review of tumors and tumor-like conditions in protozoa, coelenterata, platyhelminthes, annelida, sipunculida, and arthropods, excluding insects. In Neoplasms and related disorders of invertegrate and lower vertebrate animals. *National Cancer Institute Monograph*, 1969, *31*, 671-682.

Spector, S., Luparello, T. J., et al. Response of asthmatics to methacholine and suggestion. *American Review of Respiratory Disease*, 1976, *113*, 43-50.

Sperry, R. Mental phenomenon as casual determinants in brain function. In G. Globus (Ed.), *Brain and conscious experience*. New York: Plenum, 1976.

Sperry, R. W. Bridging science and values: a unifying review of mind and brain. *American Psychologist*, 1977, *32*, 237-245.

Spinelli, D. H., & Pribram, K. H. Changes in visual recovery functions and unit activity produced by frontal and temporal cortex stimulation. *Electroencephalography and Clinical Neurophysiology*, 1967, *22*, 143-149.

Spinelli, D. N., & Pribram, K. H. Changes in visual recovery functions produced by temporal lobe stimulation in monkeys. *Electroencephalography and Clinical Neurophysiology*, 1966, *20*, 44-49.

Spreng, L. F., Johnson, L. C., & Lubin, A. Autonomic correlates of eye movement bursts during stage REM sleep. *Psychophysiology*, 1968, *4*, 311-323.

Spring, C., Greenberg, L., Scott, J., & Hopwood, J. Electrodermal activity in hyperactive boys who are methylphenidate responders. *Psychophysiology*, 1974, *11*, 436-442.

Squires, D. F. Neoplasia in a coral? *Science*, 1965, *148*, 503-505.

Stanbury, J. B., Wyngaarden, J. B., & Fredrickson, D. S. (Eds.), *The metabolic basis of inherited disease*. New York: McGraw-Hill, 1969, 261-262.

Stapp, H. P., Bell's theorem and world progess. *Il Nuovo Cimento*, 1975, *29*, 270-276.

Stapp, H. P. S-matrix interpretation of quantum theory. *Physiological Review*, 1971, *103*, 1303-1320.

Starr, M. K. Some new fundamental considerations of variety-seeking behavior. *Behavioral Science*, 1980, *25*, 171-179.

Stein, J. J. Comments on carcinoma of the colon and rectum. *Cancer*, 1974, *34*, 799-800.

Steinberg, S. *Time*, April 17, 1978, 92-96.

Steinschneider, A., Lipton, E. L., & Richmond, J. B. Auditory sensitivity in the infant: effect of intensity on cardiac and motor responsivity. *Child Development*, 1966, *37*, 233-252.

Stern, J. A., & Janes, C. L. Personality and psychopathology. In W. F. Prokasy & D. C. Raskin (Eds.), *Electrodermal activity in psychological research*. New York: Academic Press, 1973, 283-

346.

Stern, J. A., McClure, J., & Costello, C. Depression—Assessment and ætiology. In C. Costello (Ed.), *Symptoms of psychopathology—a handbook.* New York: John Wiley & Sons, 1970, 169-200.

Stern, R. Nota sulle richerche del dottore tanchon interno la frequenza del cancro. *Ann Universali di Medicina,* 1844, *110,* 484.

Storer, E.J. The cephalic phase of gastric secretion. In J. G. Allen (Ed.), *The physiology and treatment of peptic ulcer.* Chicago: University of Chicago Press, 1959, 14-44.

Strong, L. C. *Discussion on the AAAS research conference on cancer,* 1945, 104.

Suebak, S., & Stoyva, J. High arousal can be pleasant and exciting: the theory of psychological reversals. *Biofeedback and Self-Regulation,* 1980, 5, 439-444.

Sullivan, Anne. Personal communication, June, 1973.

Sundstroem, E. S., & Michaels, G. In *Mem. University of California,* 1942, *12.*

Suss, R., Kinzel, V., & Scribner, J. (Eds.) *Cancer—Experiments and concepts.* New York: Springer-Verlag, 1973, 9-10.

Sutherland, J. *A general systems philosophy for the social and behavioral sciences.* New York: Braziller, 1973.

Szent-György, A. *Electronic biology and cancer: a new theory of cancer.* New York: Marcel Dekker, 1976.

Tanguay, P. E., Ornitz, E. M., Forsythe, A. B., & Ritvo, E. R. Rapid eye movement (REM) activity in normal and autistic children during REM sleep. *Journal of Autism and Childhood Schizophrenia,* 1976, *6,* 275-288.

Tarlau, M., & Smalheiser, I. Personality patterns in patients with malignant tumors of the breast and cervix: an exploratory study. *Psychosomatic Medicine,* 1951, *13,* 117-121.

Taylor, R. S., Carroll, B. E., & Lloyd, J. W. Mortality among women in three Catholic religious orders with special reference to cancer. *Cancer,* 1959, *12,* 1207-1225.

Ten Seldam, R. E. J. Skin cancer in Australia. National Cancer Institute Monograph No. 10. Washington, D.C. U.S. Government Printing Office, 1963, 153-166.

Tereschchenko, I. P. The state of the higher part of the central nervous system in rats during the formation and growth of induced tumors. *(Voprosy Onkologii,* 1958, *4,* 418-424.

Tereschchenko, I. P. The influence of novocaine on Brown-Pierce tumor metastases. *Vosprosy Onkologii,* 1956, *2,* 414-416.

Thomas, C. B., & Greenstreet, R. L. Psychobiological characteristics in youth as predictors of five disease states: suicide, mental illness, hypertension, coronary heart disease and tumor. *Johns Hopkins Medical Journal,* 1973, *132,* 16-43.

Thompson, W. R. *Foundations of physiological psychology.* New York: Harper & Row, 1967, 300.

Thompson, W. R. Development and the biophysical bases of personality. In E. F. Borgatta & W. W. Lambert (Eds.), *Handbook of personality theory and research.* Chicago: Rand McNally, 1968, 149-214.

Toffler, A. *The third wave.* New York: William Morrow & Co., 1980.

Toth, B. A critical review of experiments in chemical carcinogenesis using newborn animals. *Cancer Research,* 1968, *28,* 727-738.

Trainin, N. Adrenal imbalance in mouse skin carcinogenesis. *Cancer Research,* 1963, *23,* 415-419.

Trillin, A. S. Of dragons and garden peas. *New England Journal of Medicine,* 1981, *304,,* 699-701.

Tromp, S. W. The possible effect of meteorological stress on cancer and its importance for psychosomatic cancer research. *Experientia* (Basel), 1974, *30,* 1474-1478.

Turkevich, N. M. Significance of typologic characteristics of the nervous system in formation and development of cancer of the mammary gland in mice. *Voprosy Onkologii,* 1955, *1,* 64-70.

Turkevich, N. M., & Balitsky, K. Development of inoculated tumors in animals under conditions of pharmacological action on the central nervous system. *Vrachebnoe Delo,* 1953, *3,* 201-204.

Turkevich, N. M., Kunitsa, L. K., & Matveichuk, J. D. Effect of reserpine on development of induced tumor of the mammaries in rats. *Voprosy Onkologii,* 1965, *1,* 94-102.

Ukolova, M. A., Bordyushkov, Y. N., Garkavi, L. H., Goncharova, V. K., & Kvakina, H. B. The effect of direct hypothalamus stimulation on the tumour process. *Acta Unio Internationalis Contra Cancrum,* 1964, *20,* 1604-1607.

Unna, P. G. *Die histopathologie der hautkrankheiten.* Berlin: A. Hirschwald, 1894.

Urbach, F. *Anatomy and pathophysiology of skin tumor capillaries* (National Cancer Institute Monograph No. 10). Washington, D.C. U.S. Government Printing Office, 1963.

Urbach, F., Rose, D. B., & Bonnem, M. Genetic and environmental interaction in skin carcinogenesis. In *Environment and cancer.* Published for the University of Texas at Houston, M. D. Anderson Hospital and Tumor Institute, Baltimore: The Williams & Wilkins Company, 1972, 355-371.

Venables, P. H. The effect of auditory and visual stimulation on the skin potential response of schizophrenics. *Brain, A Journal of Neurology,* 1960, *83,* 77-92.

Venables, P. H. Input dysfunction in schizophrenia. In B. A. Maher (Ed.), *Progress in experimental personality research.* New York: Academic Press, 1964, 1-47.

Venables, P. H. Progress in psychophysiology: some applications in the field of abnormal psychology. In P. H. Venables & M. J. Christie (Eds.), *Research in psychophysiology.* New York: John Wiley & Sons, 1975, 418-437.

Venables, P. H. Selectivity of attention, withdrawal, and cortical activation. *Archives of General Psychiatry,* 1963, *9,* 74-78.

Venables, P. H., & Wing, J. K. Level of arousal and the subclassification of schizophrenia. *Archives of General Psychiatry,* 1962, *7,*

114-119.

Vernon, J., & McGill, T. E.   Utilization of visual stimulation during sensory deprivation. *Perceptual and Motor Skills,* 1960, *11,* 214.

von Verschuer, O., cited in Baumler, E.   *Cancer—a review of international research.* London: Queen Anne Press, 1968, 98.

Vessey, S. H.   Effects of grouping on levels of circulating antibodies in mice. *Proceedings of the Society for Experimental Biology and Medicine,* 1964, *115,* 252-255.

Vieweg, W., Reitz, R., & Weinstein, R.   Addison's disease secondary to metastatic carcinoma—an example of adrenocortical and ad-renomedullary insufficiency. *Cancer,* 1973, *31,* 1240-1243.

Vinogradova, O. S.   *The orientation reaction and its neurophysiological mechanisms.* Moscow: Academy Pedsg Sciences, (RSFSR), 1961.

Vitrey, M.   *Etude polygraphique de l'insomnie chez l'homme.* Lyon, France: Imprimerie des Beaux-Arts, J. Tixier et Fils, 1967.

Vogel, G. W., Thurmond, A., Gibbons, P., Sloan, K., Boyd, M., and Walker M.   REM sleep reduction effects on depression syndromes. *Archives of General Psychiatry,* 1975, *32,* 765-777.

Voskresenskaia, A. K.   An attempt to obtain experimental cancer in dogs and the role of the nervous system in the origin of the neoplastic process. In *Publications from the I.P. Pavlov Physiological Laboratories* (Vol. 14), 1948. (In Russian).

Wachtel, P.   Investigation and its discontents: some constraints on progress in psychological research. *American Psychologist,* 1980, *35,* 399-408.

Walker, E.   Consciousness in the quantum theory of measurement. *Journal of the Study of Consciousness,* 1972, *5,* 46-63.

Walker, E. H.   The nature of consciousness. *Mathematical Biosciences,* 1970, *7,* 131-178.

Walker, J. M., Floyd, T. C., Fein, G. et al.   Effects of exercise on sleep. *Journal of Applied Physiology,* 1978, *44,* 945-951.

Walshe, W. H.   *The nature and treatment of cancer.* London, England: Taylor and Walton, 1846.

Warburg, O.   *Uber den stoffwechsel der tumoren.* Arbeiten aus dem Kaiser Wilhelm Institut fur Biologie. Hrsg. von Otto Warburg. Berlin: J. Springer, 1926.

Warburg, O.   On the origin of cancer cells. *Science,* 1956, *123,* 309-314.

Warburg, O., Wind, F., & Negelein, E.   Metabolism of tumors in the body. *Klinische Wochenschrift,* 1926, *5,* 829-832.

Ware, J. C.   Psychophysiological arousal and subsequent sleep patterns. *Dissertation Abstracts International.* Section B. Sciences and Engineering 1976, *37,* 3125-3126.

Watanabe, T.   Regression of mouse ascites tumors by the treatment with bacterial extracts. *Japanese Journal of Experimental Medicine,* 1966, *36,* 453-455.

Watson, J. D.   *Molecular biology of the gene.* Menlo Park, California: W. A. Benjamin, Inc., 1970, 588-628.

Watts, J. W., & Fulton, J. F. Intussusception—the relation of the cerebral cortex to intestinal motility in the monkey. *New England Journal of Medicine,* 1934, *210,* 883-896.

Weale, R. A. Notes on the photometric significance of the human crystalline lens. *Vision Research,* 1961, *1,* 183-191.

Webb, W. B., & Friedman, J. Attempts to modify the sleep patterns of the rat. *Physiology and Behavior,* 1971, *6,* 459-460.

Weingarten, M., & Spinelli, D. N. Retinal receptive field changes produced by auditory and somatic stimulation. *Experimental Neurology,* 1966, *15,* 363-376.

Weiss, J. M. Somatic effects of predictable and unpredictable shock. *Psychosomatic Medicine,* 1970, *32,* 397-408.

Weiss, S., & Baker, J. P. The carotid sinus reflex in health and disease. *Medicine,* 1933, *12,* 297-354.

Wekler, W. I. Effects of age and experience on play and exploration of young chimpanzees. *Journal of Comparative and Physiological Psychology,* 1956, *49,* 223-226.

Welch, R. Personal communication, January 1980.

Weltman, A. S., Sackler, A. M., Schwartz, R., & Owen, H. Effects of isolation stress on female albino mice. *Laboratory Animal Care, 1968, 18,* 426-435.

Werder, A. A., Hardin, C. A., & Garth, R. S. Enhancement of methylcholanthrene carcinogenesis by distant surgical trauma. *Surgery,* 1959, *45,* 642-644.

West, P. M. Discussion—comparative case summaries. In J. A. Gengerelli & F. J. Kirkner (Eds.), *The psychological variables in human cancer.* Berkeley: University of California Press, 1954, 92-93.

Weybrew, B. B. *Prediction of adjustment to the Antarctic* (Technology Report 350). U.S. Naval Medical Research Laboratory, New London, Connecticut, April 1961.

White, J. E., Strudwick, W. J., Ricketts, W. N., & Sampson, C. Cancer of the skin in negroes: a review of 31 cases. *Journal of the American Medical Association,* 1961, *178,* 845-847.

White, K. L., Williams, T. F., & Greenberg, B. G. Ecology of medical care. *New England Journal of Medicine,* 1961, *265,* 885-892.

White, M. A., The social significance of mental disease. *Archives of Neurology and Psychiatry,* 1929, *22,* 873.

Wigner, E. P. Epistemology of quantum mechanics. *Psychology Issues,* 1969, *6,* 22-36.

Wigner, E. P. The place of consciousness in modern physics. In C. Muses & A. Young (Eds.), *Consciousness and reality.* New York: Avon Books, 1972, 132-149.

Wigner, E. P. *Symmetries and reflections.* Bloomington, Indiana: Indiana University Press, 1967.

Willingham, S. Personal communication, March 1981.

Wilson, C. *Mysteries.* London: Hodder & Stoughton, 1978.

Wilson, C. *The philosopher's stone.* New York: Warner Paperback Library, 1974.

Wilson, C.   New pathways in psychology.   New York: Taplinger Publishing Co., 1972.

Wilson, C.   The black room.   New York: Pyramid Books, 1971.

Wilson, C.   Poetry and mysticism.   San Francisco: City Lights Books, 1969.

Wilson, C.   Religion and the rebel.   Cambridge: Riverside Press, Houghton-Mifflin Co., 1957.

Wimsatt, W. C.   Reductionism, levels of organization and the mind-body problem.   In G. G. Globus, G.   Maxwell, & I.   Savodnik (Eds.), Consciousness and the brain.   New York: Plenum, 1976, 205-267.

Wishner, J.   The concept of efficiency in psychological health and in psychopathology.   Psychological Review, 1955, 62, 69-80.

Wistar, R., Jr., & Hildemann, W. H.   Effect of stress on transplantation immunity in mice.   Science, 1960, 131, 159-160.

Witzel, L.   Anamnese und weiterkrankungen bei patienten mit bosarteigen neubildungen.   Medizinische Klinik, 1970, 65, 876-879.

Wu, C.   Biochemical correlation of oncogenesis with ontogenesis.   International Journal of Cancer, 1973, 11, 438-447.

Wundt, W. M.   Principles of physiological psychology.   New York: The Macmillan Co., 1910.

Wynder, E. L., & Hoffman, D.   Carcinogens in the air.   In Environment and cancer (A collection of papers presented at the twenty-fourth Annual Symposium on Fundamental Cancer Research, 1971).   Baltimore: The Williams and Wilkins Company (for the M. D. Anderson Hospital and Tumor Institute in Houston, Texas), 1972, 118-138.

Wynder, E. L., & Hoffman, D.   Tobacco and tobacco smoke—Studies in experimental carcinogenesis.   New York and London: Academic Press, 1967.

Yerkes, R. M., & Dodson, J. D.   The relation of strength of stimulus to rapidity of habit formation.   Journal of Comparative Neurology and Psychology, 1908, 18, 459-482.

Young, A. M.   The reflexive universe - Evolution of consciousness.   New York: Delacorte Press, 1976.

Zubek, J. P. (Ed.)   Sensory deprivation—Fifteen years of research.   New York: Appleton-Century-Crofts, 1969.

Zuckerman, M.   Perceptual isolation as a stress situation—a review.   Archives of General Psychiatry, 1964, 11, 225-276.

Zuckerman, M.   The sensation seeking motive.   In B.   A.   Maher (Ed.), Progress in experimental personality research. New York: Academic Press, 1974, 7, 79-148.

Zuckerman, M.   Theoretical formulations.   In J. P.   Zubek (Ed.), Sensory deprivation—Fifteen years of research.   New York: Appleton-Century-Crofts, 1969, 407-433.

Zuckerman, M., & Haber, M. M.   Need for stimulation as a source of stress response to perceptual isolation.   Journal of Abnormal Psychology, 1965, 70, 371-377.

Zung, W. K., Wilson, W. P., & Dodson, W. E.   Effect of depressive disorders on sleep EEG responses.   Archives of General Psychiatry, 1964, 10, 439-445.

Index

Sex hormones, and carcinogenesis, 12, 90, 102
Sexual activity, as deautomatization, 147
Sexual behavior disorder, boredom as one cause of, 146–147
Skin cancer:
  in blacks, 87–88
  and exposure to sunlight, 87–88
  and polycyclic hydrocarbons, 166
  posited mismatch condition contributing to, 106
  See also Cancer; Carcinogenesis
Sleep:
  anti-depressant therapy and, 142
  and cancer interrelations, 107–108
  as end result of automatization of attention, 40, 142–143
  in gerontological populations, 140
  gastroesophageal reflux and, 146
  headaches exacerbated by, 145–146
  and lesions of posterior hypothalamus, 121
  parasympathetic activation and, 145
  in primary depression, 141–142
  and pro-inflammatory hormones, 70
  and sensory stimulation, 137–138
  tonic and phasic events, as information/control mechanisms, 28–32
  and trophotropic system, 121
  See also Automatization; Boredom; REM density; REM deprivation; REM sleep
Sleep apnea:
  in asymptomatic older males, 144
  attenuation of, by rocking bed, 143
  and boredom, 143–144
  and excessive daytime sleepiness, 142–144
  homeostatic aspects of, 143–144
  obstructive, characteristics of, 143
  obstructive, and weight gain, 143
  as partial sleep deprivation for depression, 143–144
  posited homeostatic function of, 144
  as reflective of generalized systemic

entropy or deautomatization, 144
Sleep deprivation:
  and amelioration of depression, 142
  apnea as effecting homeostatic and heterostatic, 143–144
  posited effects of, on carcinogenesis, 107
  See also Sleep; REM deprivation
Sleep disorders:
  as compensatory information augmenting mechanisms, 137–146
  posited interrelations with carcinogenesis, 107–108
  See also Insomnia; Parasomnias; Narcolepsy; Sleep apnea
Sleep latency, in hyperactive children, 40
Sleep walking-talking, as compensatory information augmenting mechanism, 145
Sperry, R., 157, 161
Sponge, absence of carcinogenesis in, 64
Spontaneous remission, 165
Sporting events, as deautomatization, 171
Stimulant drugs:
  high doses, as promotors of cancer, 67–68
  as inhibitory to cancer, 67–69
  long term maladaptive effects of, 128
  paradoxical relaxing effect of, 26, 128
Stimulation:
  of anterior hypothalamus, and autonomic balance, 72–73
  of frontal cortex, effects on information processing rate in CNS, 73
  of posterior cortex, effects of, on information processing rates in CNS, 73
  of posterior hypothalamus, and autonomic balance, 72–73
  of posterior hypothalamus, and cancer regression, 73